TREATING FOOD ALLERGY

My Way!

*Exploring the Most Important
Food Allergies*

TREATING FOOD ALLERGY

My Way!

Exploring the Most Important Food Allergies

William E. Walsh, M.D.

with contributions by
Denise and Peter Zang

ACA Publications, Inc.
St. Paul, Minnesota

International Standard Book Number 0-9631544-3-5
Library of Congress Catalog Card Number TXU494777

Designed and Composed by Barbara Field
Printed by Viking Press Inc.

ACA Publications, Inc.
1690 University Avenue West, Suite 450
St. Paul, Minnesota 55104

Printed in the United States of America

Contents

Preface

When we go on a journey, we expect to complete it safely and at our destination. Unfortunately, that doesn't always happen. Think of the poor passengers on the Titanic who paid their money to enjoy the maiden voyage of this luxurious ocean liner, content in the knowledge that the ship was virtually unsinkable. Unfortunately, this bold claim made no impression on the iceberg that brought their voyage to disaster.

Fortunately, most of the time our journeys end safely and we reach our destination, usually with the help of a few key people. For instance, if you were going to Germany you might first visit a travel agent, an expert in trip planning. To get to the airport you call a cab; the driver is an expert in city transportation. You board a plane whose pilot is an expert in flying. You stay in a hotel staffed by experts in lodging. Your trip goes smoothly because competent experts handle each step.

A book is like a journey for your mind. You read it because you have a destination or goal you want to reach; when you finish, you hope to have reached this goal. If the book is a detective story or science fiction novel, you want excitement and entertainment; from a biography or wildlife novel, you desire knowledge and adventure. From a medical book, you hope to gain the most precious knowledge of all, a way to improve your health.

That is the purpose of this book. I hope that when you complete your journey through its pages, you gain a little knowledge to ease the problems life makes you face. And just as you have every right to question the qualifications of the people who help you on your make-believe trip to Germany, you have every right to question my qualifications, since I am your travel guide, cabby, and pilot on this trip. Let me give them to you.

I am a medical doctor with the same M.D. degree as a pediatrician, family doctor, or internist. After completing medical school, I served two years in the U.S. Air Force, where I had the opportunity to care for an allergy clinic. The field of allergy fascinated me, and I realized I would be happy spending my life treating people with allergy problems; I also realized that the field is so complicated I needed further training. As I think back to those days, I know I was right in both cases. I am happy treating people with allergy and I'm glad I sought further training to put me on firmer ground in this demanding field.

This training was obtained at the Mayo Clinic, where I spent four hard-working but enjoyable years. The clinic, through its expert teaching staff and diverse patient load, offers the allergist-in-training magnificent opportunities to study the many areas he or she is responsible for when treating people, areas such as allergic dermatology, allergic chest disease, allergic gastrointestinal disease, and many others, as well as how pollen, dust, and mold affect patients with allergy.

After completing my training at the Mayo Clinic, I moved to St. Paul, Minnesota, in 1970, where I started my current allergy practice. Shortly afterward, I took and passed an examination certifying me as a specialist in allergy. The certificate is from the American Board of Allergy and Immunology and is recognized by the American Board of Pediatrics and the American Board of Internal Medicine.

The American Board of Allergy and Immunology sponsors active programs to keep allergists up to date, including providing the opportunity to retake the test at specified intervals, a process called voluntary recertification. To ensure that my knowledge remained current, I took the recertification exam in 1980 and again in 1990, on each occasion earning my recertification diploma.

I have described my credentials to assure you that the book you are reading was written by a qualified medical doctor who tries to stay current with modern scientific knowledge of allergic illness. Although the training and diplomas are essential to making a medical book credible, they are only part of the reason this book exists. Equally important are several other factors.

One factor is perhaps most significant because it makes me uniquely qualified to write this book. I share with many people a great susceptibility to the harm caused by foods. Perhaps that's understandable; who wouldn't be fascinated by a medical illness if they were its victim? I know my medical problems steered me toward my specialty in the first place, and I remember how it happened.

I was walking to work on a lovely fall day in 1965, looking quite nice in my spiffy Air Force captain's uniform. But my mind wasn't on enjoying the warm, green Nebraska scenery; instead my thoughts twisted and turned as I considered the many specialized fields of medicine my M.D. degree unlocked. Which one for me? Should it be Family Medicine, which brings with it the satisfaction of caring for all the illnesses of my patients, of being the first doctor they call when they are ill? Or maybe Obstetrics, for the joy of delivering healthy babies? Or perhaps Plastic Surgery, for the pride of restoring a ravished face? Or Psychiatry, with its awesome potential for working with the human mind and emotions?

Then the obvious struck me, and I stopped and laughed. There I was, standing in a green and weedy field at the height of the fall ragweed pollen season, my eyes running like a crying baby's and my nose dripping like old plumbing with a leak, wheezing like a couch potato running a marathon. To add to my miseries, my armpits were itching from contact dermatitis caused by sensitivity to a deodorant. I said to myself, "Bill, whatever could you be other then an allergist?"

I have never regretted that decision, and as I pick up new allergies, they serve to reinforce and renew my interest in, and fascination for, the field of allergy. When foods began to trouble me, my attention to food allergy increased enormously, especially when articles in the allergy literature started questioning whether allergists paid enough attention to patient's complaints about food. I discovered I paid little attention, and I resolved to change.

Eating when hungry, drinking when thirsty, and making resolutions are equally easy; growing food in a drought, finding water in a desert, and keeping resolutions are equally hard. However, because of my own food reactions, keeping my resolve to study food allergy was easy. Unfortunately I found treating food allergy uncommonly difficult. Why? Because my patients told me about food reactions that the allergy literature said weren't supposed to happen, reactions to foods the literature said didn't cause symptoms. In fact, because my patients' stories of their food allergies contradicted the allergy literature, I was becoming more and more confused and frustrated.

That I needed to learn about food allergy was obvious; what was not obvious was where this knowledge existed. I was forced to choose between accepting the allergy literature's view of food allergy or believing my patients when they told me their weird-sounding stories of food reactions. I chose to believe my patients.

I'm glad I did. Over a period of years, their strange tales started to make sense, a pattern of reactions emerged, a dietary approach was born. I wish I could say the diet sprang from my brilliant deductions, but that's not true. My patients taught me the diet a little at a time as they related their discoveries about the foods that aggravated their headaches, hives, and diarrhea. Each discovery lessened the confusion surrounding food allergy; each discovery added another important element to the diet.

Which brings me to the factor prompting me to launch this book at this time. My dietary approach is ready. The diet works for a great many of my patients, and it's time for me to organize the information more completely.

That's why I'm writing this book.

Acknowledgments

This book and the diet it describes would not exist without the help of many contributors. I am honored to acknowledge this help and to thank those whose generous assistance was so essential.

Much of the dietary advice contained in this book is new and surprising and was originally discovered, not by me, but by patients observant enough to recognize the foods and beverages responsible for their illnesses. These novel aspects of the diet became permanent additions when other patients found they were important in controlling their symptoms.

To those patients whose insights shaped the diet and to those patients who followed the diet and confirmed its value, I extend a heartfelt thank you. It would never have been developed without your counsel and guidance.

Just as the help of my patients was essential in developing this diet, so was the assistance of the nurses who work with me. Each is a registered nurse who has specialized for many years in the care of the allergic patient. My nurses and I approach the treatment our allergic patients as a team, from initial evaluation and diagnosis through followup care. I want to express my gratitude to each member of that team: Shirley Hess, Arleene Nietz, Corinne Peterson, Jan Ryan, and Caryl Steenberg.

I am also grateful for the fine work and cooperation of Denise and Peter Zang. Peter's expertise as a chef is truly appreciated. He and Denise supplied recipes to help our patients prepare foods that are acceptable on the diet. Denise was also of great help in writing this book, especially the last few chapters.

Many others have contributed to the diet and the book, including Barbara Field, whose skills with writing helped make sense of many murky passages. To all of you, my deepest thanks.

The case histories described in this book are representative of many conversations with patients who have similar illnesses and food allergies. They are included to help the reader understand food allergy and its treatment. Although the essence of each case history is preserved, the names, occupations, and certain facts have been changed to prevent recognition of the patients and protect their privacy.

The Key

Were you ever out walking alone, late at night, the wind blowing icy needles of rain against your face, the darkness closing in around you. Chilled and uncomfortable, your imagination populates the night with vague and sinister demons. An uneasiness lurks at the edges of your consciousness, a wariness that raises the hair at the back of your neck, a sensation that you're being watched. At last you see the familiar sight of home, a safe haven with its bright lights and warm, dry rooms smiling a welcome that says, "Come in and I will give you comfort and protect you from the dark night." With a great feeling of relief you reach into your pocket and find—no key! You are left out in the cold, damp night.

Such is the importance of a key in our lives; it allows us to enter locked places that assure us warmth and protection. A key is equally important in our thinking. A branch of knowledge may be as elementary as the techniques used in digging a hole or as esoteric as the formulas used in flying to the moon. But whether simple or complicated, the process of thinking depends on certain key facts so important that if they were missing, the branch of knowledge would be reduced to confusion and uncertainty.

1

And so it is with medicine. Over the centuries many areas of medicical knowledge advanced dramatically when certain key facts became known. Just think of the wonderful heart, lung, and kidney transplants performed today—procedures previous generations of doctors couldn't even imagine—or the fantastic antibiotics that routinely kill germs that used to send us to the grave. Truly remarkable advances due to the discovery of a few key facts.

Unfortunately, not all areas of medicine have experienced such dramatic advances. One area of medical knowledge that has made little gain is the science of food allergy. Food allergy remains mired in confusion and uncertainty because the scientists who study it and the doctors who treat it are missing a crucial piece of information—information so vital that without it, treatment usually ends in failure. In this book we will examine that key piece of information, how a remarkably common group of foods and beverages can cause so many illnesses in so many people.

How To Use This Book

Don't Try To Make This Book Your Doctor

The purpose of this book is to tell you about the way I treat food allergy. I hope to alert you to some of the foods and beverages that cause my patients' symptoms—they may also hurt you. If so, and if you avoid them, I hope you will stop hurting. I did not write this book to tell you how to diagnose these illnesses. This diagnosis must be done by your primary doctor, who may be a family doctor, pediatrician, or internist. That is their specialty.

In my allergy practice, I try to make sure each of my patients has a primary doctor who has already diagnosed allergy and excluded—as far as possible—nonallergic illness as the cause of my patients' symptoms. If you were my patient and we questioned the cause of your illness, I would send you to your primary doctor for diagnosis. Go to him or her now if there is any question about your diagnosis. Don't try to guess your diagnosis by reading this book.

If your doctor wants help in diagnosis, he or she may suggest you see a neurologist, dermatologist, or other specialist; if so, for heaven's sake, take this advice. Don't try to make this book your diagnostic specialist.

Maintain a Healthy Diet While You Follow My Dietary Advice

Some of the foods and beverages I ask you to avoid add no value to a healthy diet. Other foods and beverages are championed by dietary experts who teach us they are a necessary part of a healthy diet (a number of dieticians are scandalized that we ask our patients to exclude them). Excluding these foods and beverages is not fatal to a healthy diet. There are plenty of healthy foods you can eat while you follow my diet.

In certain circumstances, there is a danger you will slip into a nutritionally inadequate and therefore unhealthy diet. For instance, if you already follow a medically pre-scribed diet that excludes healthy foods, and you also try to exclude the foods and beverages that trouble my patients, your diet may be inadequate and your health threatened. The same threat could surface with a diet not prescribed by a doctor. *If there is any chance your diet will become inadequate and unhealthy, do not follow my diet until you consult your doctor or a dietician.*

Why

As humans, we become uneasy and irritated when forced to follow instructions and we don't understand why. Who can blame us for this desire for knowledge, this demand to have *why* explained to us. Perhaps it is this curiosity about reasons, which prompts our irritation when we are ignorant, that distinguishes humans from animals. (In distinguishing humans from animals, it sometimes helps to have clues.)

I know I share this desire to know why. When I began to realize the complexity of food allergy, it became apparent that my patients would be forced to avoid a surprising number of foods and beverages, and I didn't have any idea why this was so; what made these seemingly different foods and beverages cause the same misery? The foods and beverages are different—orange juice differs from diet pop and cheese is not the same as soy sauce—but they are also similar in their effects. Orange juice, diet pop, cheese, and soy sauce all cause the same headaches or hives or diarrhea. I was learning how to treat my food-sensitive patients, but I was not learning why my treatment worked. I was irritated and frustrated.

5

The Usual Explanation of Food Allergy

There is an explanation of food allergy that is widely accepted by allergists. All animal- and vegetable-derived foods are made up of proteins, fats, and carbohydrates. Many of the food proteins are identical to our own body's protein, and the allergic person absorbs and digests them with no difficulty. But some proteins are different. They are only found in such foods as shrimp or nuts or cows' milk. The body does not recognize them, and in the allergic person these strange proteins lead to trouble.

When even a tiny amount of the strange shrimp, nut, or milk protein gains entrance into the allergic person's bloodstream, it is grabbed by an antibody called IgE. This antibody alerts the body to the presence of the strange protein, and the body reacts alarmingly. It releases chemicals that welt the skin in hives, clamp down on the small air passages in the lungs, causing wheezing, and the large air passages, causing choking, and dilate the blood vessels, dropping the blood pressure and threatening shock and unconsciousness.

This is an irrational overreaction to a harmless protein, like shooting a mosquito off your leg with a shotgun. Unfortunately, the allergic person is stuck with it.

My patients were not describing this sort of food allergy. Their symptoms weren't quick, striking, and dramatic; they were chronic and persistent. Also, tiny amounts didn't set off symptoms, only excess amounts—overloads. And proteins weren't involved. Our concepts of food allergy did not fit. I was confused.

A New Type of Food Allergy

Then I recalled some principles of biochemistry I learned in medical school and an explanation became apparent. I don't know if the explanation is correct, but I think it is; I know it helped me understand why my patients need to avoid certain foods and beverages.

To understand the explanation, it helps to compare your body's cells to miniature cities. They are special cities, not at all like our present-day metropolises that use coal, oil, and natural gas for power. Instead, the cell cities in our bodies use a miracle fuel as powerful as nuclear fuel but without many of the dangers associated with nuclear power plants. (That's obvious! Have you ever heard of a cell with lead or cement shielding?)

This marvelous fuel has to be handled carefully. Instead of being shoveled or pumped into a furnace to be consumed by fire all at once, it goes through a series of furnaces, each furnace releasing energy to the cell by burning only part of the fuel. When the last furnace is done, the remaining fuel is renewed by adding special chemicals, and the whole cycle of energy production starts again. A complicated process to produce power, but tremendously efficient.

Because this energy-producing process is complicated, it needs to be controlled. In our make-believe world of the cell city, this control is achieved using methods like those of our real cities; a bureaucracy rules. Let's look at this bureaucracy.

The bureaucrats are surprisingly alike. As children they were pudgy; their classmates called them Fats or Wart or Bumble; they were the type of student who told the teacher, "The homework assignments are due today," and they never got dirty. They were perfect children, although a tad slow in their thinking, a mite short on creativity, and a bit lacking in flexibility. Anything out of the ordinary flustered them and led to confused inactivity.

As adults, the bureaucrats still are surprisingly alike. Their fellow rulers call them Robert, Alexander, and William (their exaggerated sense of importance allows no nicknames). They are pudgy, pompous, and persnickety, and good administrators as long as everything is going well; but any disruption causes disaster. You see, they are still a tad slow in their thinking, a mite short on creativity, and a bit lacking in flexibility. The bureaucracy of the cell city is unlike that of our modern society, where flexibility, creativity, and clear thought are so necessary and practical.

An old expression tells us that into every life a little rain must fall. Unfortunately for our bureaucrats, rain can turn to a flood. The problem arises from another group that populates our little cell city—an antibureaucratic group. A group of rebels.

Markedly different from the bureaucrats, this second group went by the nicknames of Sly, Speed, and Flash as youngsters; their names fit their mischief. They never finished their homework on time, so when the little bureaucrats reminded the teacher the assignments were due, they seethed with anger.

Sly, Speed, and Flash and their friends thought fast, found creativity a snap, and were utterly flexible. Unfortunately, they were also little devils. If there was trouble brewing, they were first in line. If teacher sat on a pin, their pleas of innocence rang through the room. If someone tripped a little bureaucrat, they were guilty. Engaging little chaps, but in their bodies not one grain of responsibility.

As adults, they are just as fast-thinking, creative, and flexible, and just as lacking in responsibility. Their delight and pleasure in life is to torment the bureaucrats, and they know a perfect way to achieve this fiendish goal. You see, this fantastic energy production can only work if the fuel, which is hot and corrosive, is slowly and precisely transported to the furnaces (one of the few virtues of the bureaucrats is their precision—and they are slow). Our rebels delight in sending extra trainloads of fuel to the furnaces, where they dump it all over the floor.

You can imagine what happens next. Our poor bureaucrats, faced with this mess, call out the National Guard and enlist workers from factories and offices to shovel up the corrosive goo. This makes everybody unhappy. The

National Guard is grumpy because the gooey fuel eats through their shiny boots. The office and factory workers hate the backbreaking work and their union strikes in protest, closing the assembly lines, supermarkets, and sales organizations of the little cell city. The city grinds to a halt, the voters complain, the mayor screams, the bureaucrats are reduced to quivering ineptness. It's a real mess.

Pity the poor bureaucrats. Slow-thinking, lacking creativity and flexibility, they are unprepared for this major disaster. After undergoing psychiatric treatment for acute anxiety, induced by the disruption in their precious orderliness and the upheaval in the city they rule, they slowly and ploddingly restore the energy-producing system to normal and restart the offices and factories. And calm the mayor and soothe the voters. And wait for the next onslaught of excess fuel for the furnaces.

The Moral of the Story

Perhaps you think the story of the little cell city is preposterous? Are you saying to yourself, "No way is that story a model of the cell"? If these are your thoughts, you are wrong.

What We Know

The marvelous material that stores the energy of the atom without the dangers of its radioactivity is sugar. The analogy of the furnaces is a good one; sugar slowly releases its fantastic energy, a bit at a time, as if it were traveling from furnace to furnace. In biochemistry books, this process is called the Krebs cycle or the tricarboxylic acid cycle.

The counterparts of the bureaucrats in the body are the enzymes that precisely regulate sugar's energy release. Made of proteins, the prime function of these tricky molecules in energy production is to regulate and assist in the splitting of the sugar molecule that releases energy. Without them, sugar would need furnace heat to split, making life impossible unless we were built like your home furnace. (Imagine dating someone who looks like your furnace!)

So the furnace-like production of energy actually takes place in the body; because it is regulated by enzymes, there is no need for furnace heat. Enzymes do fantastic work, but don't be fooled. They are not creative or flexible or quick thinking; they ploddingly and persistently perform the limited tasks to which they are assigned.

What I Believe To Be True

To continue the explanation, you must accept the rest of the story as I see it and believe it to be true.

It is tempting to look at our modern world, to see computers, bullet trains, and swept-wing fighter planes, and to conclude that not only has the world changed, we've changed. In some ways, perhaps we have. But not our bodies nor our cells.

The last thousand years have brought profound changes in our lifestyle. However, a thousand years is a tiny moment in the evolution of our bodies, of our cells. They are the same cells our ancestors possessed in the ancient past, in a cave, crowded close to a fire. In fact, they are not much changed from that monkey-like creature whose descendants walked upright and learned to talk. We share the same nutrition needs, digestion limits, and energy production method.

What has changed is our diet, specifically our use of refined foods. Prior to modern agriculture, foods were made of unrefined protein, starch, and fat. We all know the ponderous impact of refined fats on our bathroom scales.

Starches are made of sugar molecules, tightly bound together like links on a chain. In digestion, the individual sugars are snapped off the chain slowly and ploddingly, allowing lots of time to process each sugar and insert it into the energy production system. No hurry, everything orderly. The bureaucratic control of energy is content.

Proteins are like starches, chains of amino acids that are broken off the chain slowly, ploddingly, and contentedly.

Refining starches and proteins produces regrettable consequences. Refining breaks the bonds between sugar molecules so the sugar you eat and drink enters the stomach no longer in chains. The molecules are like the links of a busted chain; they are free. The body gobbles up this unchained sugar like a hungry shark in a goldfish aquarium. Unfortunately, although our digestion system can regulate its intake of sugar from starch, it has inadequate ability to regulate its intake of refined sugar. Conditioned by millions of years of evolution to handle a diet of starches, its enzymes do not have the flexibility and creativity to adapt to a diet high in refined sugar.

The refined sugar floods the body, causing the various systems that process sugar to overload. What happens then is unclear, although I like my fanciful explanation of the little cell city and the havoc that overload causes. I believe it has illness-causing effects, and I hope to further explain this belief in other sections of this book.

Before ending this chapter, a word about proteins. The story is much the same as with sugar. Refining breaks apart the linked amino acids that make protein. The free amino acids gush into the body, overwhelming the amino acid handling systems. The body suffers harm.

What Is Allergy?
What Is an Allergist?

Most of us became familiar with the word *allergy* as young children, either because we ourselves had an allergic reaction such as hives or eczema, or one of our siblings or friends had allergies. In other words, our understanding of allergy is based on what it *does* to people rather than what it *is*. However, before we can understand what an allergist is, we will need a more precise definition of allergy.

What Is Allergy?

Allergic illness arises from the body's sensitivity to the pollen, dust, mold, food, and certain other substances we are exposed to in the environment. Why does the body react? Because it mistakes things free of harm for things full of danger.

For instance, a harmless bit of ragweed pollen meanders by, minding its own business, not a nasty thought in its tiny mind. For some odd reason, the nose reacts fearfully to contact with this innocent pollen, rushing into frenzied activity—sneezing, dripping, itching, and stuffing up—as if the pollen were intent on starting a horrible infection. It's not—the nose is mistaken. Unfortunately, the miserable person attached to the nose suffers.

It is the same with food allergy. The wretched person affected by this process eats a little shrimp and disaster strikes. His eyes water, his body swells, he chokes as his air passages close, and his skin grows a crop of red splotches as if a heavenly painter has spattered him with barn paint. Again, a mistake in identification. The body thought the shrimp was an attacking enemy. Most uncomfortable and definitely dangerous. (It's beyond me why the body defends itself by almost killing itself!)

Pollen, dust, mold, and food do not directly cause any allergic symptoms. They are triggering mechanisms, just like the trigger on a gun. The bullets they release are numerous natural body chemicals, some with familiar names such as histamine, others with improbable names like the slow-reacting substance of anaphylaxis. These chemicals flood the body, dilating blood vessels, leaking fluid, itching nerve fibers, and, in general, making a horrible mess. They stuff the nose and hive the skin when we allergic people encounter ragweed, shrimp, and the numerous other things that cause allergies.

The Scope of Allergy

That a patient is suffering from an allergic illness is sometimes quite obvious. It may strike dramatically and quickly—the sneezing and swollen eyes after contact with ragweed and cat dander are obvious, as are the acute hives and choking after eating shrimp. The diagnosis is often confirmed by blood tests that measure an antibody, called IgE, which attaches to the ragweed, cat dander, or shrimp. Usually the skin tests are positive, again confirming the diagnosis. These reactions are within the scope of allergy.

But the allergic basis of some illnesses is not obvious. These illnesses don't strike suddenly; they develop slowly. No IgE antibody against the cause floats in the bloodstream; a skin test answer doesn't magically appear in thirty minutes. However, they also fit within the scope of allergy—they are caused by the same environmental exposures and foods that bring on the more easily recognized sudden symptoms.

Patients often fail to realize that their discomfort and pain are caused or influenced by allergy if the symptoms develop slowly, symptoms such as headache and asthma and eczema, plus many others. In fact, they frequently tell me, "I would have come to see you long ago if I had known my headaches (or chronic diarrhea or chronic hives, etc.) were due to allergy."

Two Types of Food Allergy

Food allergy frequently appears in a quickly developing form where the cause is usually obvious (i.e., a shrimp reaction). It can also appear as a slow-developing illness that is hard to diagnose.

With the sudden onset type of food allergy, people are reacting to something in the diet. Usually it is a protein, one so different from a person's own body proteins that the body becomes alarmed. For instance, there are proteins in nuts, cows' milk, and shrimp that are different from the protein making up the body's muscles and internal organs. When the body recognizes this strange protein, it triggers the allergic illness—hives, asthma, hay fever, etc. Often tiny amounts of these proteins lead to dangerous and sometimes life-threatening reactions.

But foreign protein is not the only cause of food allergy. Some food chemicals that are not protein and not foreign to the body are also involved—chemicals that live in every cell in the body, chemicals essential for metabolism, chemicals necessary for life.

Tiny amounts of these chemicals do not cause harm. Only large amounts do, quantities so sizable the body can't handle them. The illnesses caused by this type of food allergy develop slowly and the patient has a hard time identifying the guilty foods.

To unravel the mystery surrounding the diagnosis and treatment of food allergy, the harm caused by excesses of these chemicals must be recognized. We will attempt to do this as we examine food allergy more closely.

The Role of the Allergist

"Well," you ask, "what is the role of the allergist? Certainly a gastroenterologist can uncover the foods that are causing cramps and diarrhea, a neurologist can investigate foods that are provoking headaches, a dermatologist can determine the foods that are inducing hives and eczema."

Yes, they can, and they should try to find them. However, an allergist possesses unique tools and training. For example, an allergist is trained in the application and interpretation of skin tests; in diagnosing food allergy, these tests are often essential.

In drafting their majestic plan for humanity's allergies, the architects forgot to limit food allergy to one food, but allowed a rascal assistant to guarantee that many patients' food allergies involve multiple foods. Unfortunately, this makes diagnosing reactions to these multiple foods difficult or impossible without the help of food skin tests. In many cases, a doctor trying to diagnose a complicated case of food allergy without the aid of food skin tests is like a traveler without a compass—lost in a fog of uncertainty. Food skin tests, the primary tool of the allergist, often help cut through the fog.

Two examples spring easily to mind. Jimmy, an eleven-year-old patient of mine, had a particularly baffling case of asthma—darned if I could figure it out. Food allergy didn't seem to be at fault because his asthma was so persistent. He wheezed every day and his asthma didn't vary with his diet. Out of frustration, and because I didn't know how else to find the cause, we skin tested him to foods, and a large wheat reaction surfaced. I couldn't believe it! In my experience, asthma due to wheat is rare. I was surprised when, on Jimmy's next visit, his father told me the test must have been correct because Jimmy wheezed every time he ate wheat. Avoiding wheat gratifyingly calmed his asthma.

Then there is Tammy, a clerk for a local department store, who had persistent hives due to multiple foods, including such traditional ones as lettuce, celery, and carrots. If they hadn't revealed themselves on skin tests, I don't know how I would have discovered them, and Tammy's skin would still be itchy and blotchy.

Many other illustrative cases tumble around in my memory, but I believe these two serve to make the point.

To complicate matters even further, not only do allergic patients have multiple food allergies, they also have multiple allergic illnesses. In my practice, that is not the exception, it's the rule. Again, a few examples to help you understand.

Jack is a twenty-five-year-old pipefitter who often works in dusty areas that make his constantly stuffy nose shut down completely. When he visits his girlfriend in her musty basement apartment, he wheezes and his eyes swell, perhaps due to the apartment's mold, or maybe to her cat. As a toddler, cramps and diarrhea made him scream with pain and his parents' nights seem to last centuries as they listened to his suffering. As an adult, he won't eat in a restaurant because he almost strangles if a careless food handler allows a little shrimp into his food. Even avoiding shrimp isn't enough. Once or twice a week some unknown foods or beverages give him cramps and diarrhea. He's really uncomfortable.

How can Jack find out about the cat, mold, and food allergies that plague him? It is inefficient and impractical to expect Jack to see an ophthalmologist for his eyes, an otolaryngologist for his nose, a pulmonologist for his asthma, and a gastroenterologist for his diarrhea and have each of them administer a separate set of skin tests. A far more sensible approach to diagnosing the causes of Jack's nose, eye, chest, and abdominal illnesses is to send him to a doctor acceptable to all these specialists—an allergist.

I don't mean to disparage the other specialists I mentioned. Each has a role to play in good patient care. When a patient has any illness, he or she should first see a primary doctor for diagnosis and treatment and be referred to other specialists if the primary doctor wants their help. When the primary doctor suspects allergy and wants help in diagnosing the allergic causes of a patient's illness, an allergist should be consulted.

But what about the patient who has only one allergic illness such as diarrhea? Perhaps the allergist's help is not so essential, and testing by the gastroenterologist would be sufficient. Maybe, but don't forget our impish assistant architect. I guess it wasn't in his plan for the allergic patient to have only one illness.

I am reminded of Mary, a fifteen-year-old who first came to see me ten years ago, accompanied by her mother Theresa. Poor Mary had daily cramps and weekly diarrhea, which we found was due to a number of common offenders, including tomato products, citrus fruits, and beef (surprisingly, because beef is rarely a cause of diarrhea). Three years later she returned with severe hay fever, which we found was caused by oak and ragweed pollen. Mary is now married with two lovely children, whom I met when she returned recently to tell me of her asthma, probably provoked by her basement apartment's mustiness.

The moral of Mary's story? There is no way to predict that a person will always have only one allergy. Mary would have felt ridiculous returning to a gastroenterologist to explore the cause of her hay fever or asthma. Returning to an allergist made more sense.

I told you about these patients, not to glorify the allergist, but to attempt to explain the allergist's role among the specialists your primary doctor may want you to visit. I view the allergist's primary function as that of an investigator into the causes of environmental and food reactions that can affect many areas of the body and involve any specialty from dermatology to pulmonology.

It is my hope that these examples will also help you understand this complicated field of allergy, which attempts the awesome task of studying the myriad environmental agents and foods that cause diverse illnesses. I say awesome task because the troublemaker assistant architect of allergy had no more pity on the *doctor* diagnosing allergy then he had on the miserable *sufferer*. Multiple environmental agents (dust, mold, pollen, animals), multiple foods, and multiple illnesses are often as difficult (and sometimes impossible) for the doctor to *diagnose* as they are for the patient to *tolerate*.

The complexity of allergy makes diagnosis difficult and, in my opinion, creates the need for the specialty of allergy—men and women specifically trained to recognize and test for the multiple illnesses caused by the environment, by foods, and as you will see later, by food additives.

Overview of Food Allergy

The ways in which people react to foods vary as much as the ways in which they comb their hair. They can react quickly and dramatically and recover equally rapidly—or become sick slowly and recover sluggishly. One food or many foods may bring pain and discomfort. The involved foods can be obvious and the patient sure of the cause, or the foods obscure and the person confused. For some, food allergies strike when they consume even a minuscule amount; others need to eat or drink a comparatively large quantity before experiencing pain and discomfort. On skin testing, the harmful foods may surface, or perversely hide their identity. Complicated for these poor people, isn't it?

Sudden, Dramatic Food Reactions

For many people, even tiny amounts of such foods as nuts, fish, peanuts, and shellfish can precipitate severe and life-threatening illnesses; because they are quick-striking and dramatic, a person's attention is immediately drawn to the food. There is usually no difficulty in determining the culprit. The only treatment for this type of food allergy is avoidance—don't eat the offending food.

An example of someone with this type of allergy is the person who dines at a nice restaurant, enjoying a delectable meal of shrimp. Suddenly his eyes swell and tears flow, his nasal passages become blocked, his skin erupts with angry red hives, and the swelling in his air passages begins to strangle him. The reaction is dramatic, frightening, and dangerous. No more shrimp!

Sometimes the severe reaction occurs during or after a meal at which many foods are eaten. If the multiple foods consumed make it difficult to identify the dangerous food, blood tests or careful skin tests to food will often unmask the offender.

The Single Food Allergy

The quickness and severity of dangerous food reactions usually point directly to the involved food. Another aid to diagnosis arises when a person reacts to a single food. This is especially helpful when the ill effects appear shortly after the food is eaten. If you have diarrhea or hives every time you eat corn or carrots, you know where the problem lies.

Sometimes, a commonly consumed food such as wheat, or a beverage such as milk, is at fault. Because the food is eaten at every meal, it's hard to pinpoint (infrequently consumed foods are easier). If the patient has a hunch corn or milk provokes symptoms, he or she can avoid the suspect food or beverage for a week and then reintroduce it to the diet—repeatedly if necessary—and the waxing and waning of symptoms will usually confirm the suspicion. If there is still doubt, a skin test will often provide certainty.

Multiple Food Allergies

Now the diagnosis becomes more difficult. As the number of foods causing symptoms multiplies, the difficulty in finding these foods also multiplies. When a person eats or drinks a number of potentially harmful foods at each meal, it is easy to be confused. Although it is *unusual* for the patient with one food allergy to pursue allergy consultation, it is usually *necessary* for the patient with many food allergies to seek help.

Many examples come to mind, including Genny, a fifty-five-year-old mother of four and grandmother of three whose internist sent her to me after years of struggling unsuccessfully to treat her daily abdominal pains and crippling migraine headaches. Her symptoms began after her second child was born and often made the demanding role of motherhood a dreadful ordeal. In fact, pain often forced her to take to her bed, even when her children were small and needed supervision. She was miserable.

When we skin tested Genny her back flared with hives to every food tested—clearly she had multiple and serious food allergies. When I considered how to treat her, I admit I was discouraged. However, we pursued our usual approach to the patient with multiple food allergies: change the environment to reduce pollen, dust, animal, and mold exposures so she could have more "room" for food allergy; guide her in avoiding the worst foods and beverages; persuade her to rotate the rest of the foods in her diet frequently.

It worked! Genny returned to see me in three months with both abdominal pain and migraines markedly improved. No days spent in bed. My staff and I were delighted.

There are many people like Genny in our practice, each with his or her own pitiful tale. With each patient I worry whether I will be able to control these truly troublesome multiple food allergies; with almost all patients I find the tools of the allergist—combined with the patient's fine cooperation and hard work—bring about a pleasing reduction of miserable symptoms.

Slow-Developing Food Reactions

Now the diagnosis of food allergy becomes even more difficult. We no longer have the guidance of the fast-striking food reaction (i.e., eat shrimp, get sick immediately). To further confuse diagnosis, most of the patients in my practice with slow-developing food allergies are allergic to multiple foods with all the puzzlement that multiple food allergy introduces.

For instance, Linda is a forty-two-year-old printing salesperson who must often entertain her clients at restaurants. She never develops symptoms after dinner, but the next morning she wakes up feeling crummy. She feels bloated and her bathroom scale agrees; her cramps and diarrhea force her to stay home from the office or to try to go to work and have a miserable day; she is tired, irritable, and understandably depressed. (Anyone who wakes up feeling like Linda does would be depressed.)

Linda came to see me because she couldn't figure out why eating out caused such severe symptoms. She is a bright woman—any salesperson needs to be sharp to be successful—so it wasn't lack of mental ability that prevented her from recognizing the cause of her problem. The harmful foods were concealed because they were *multiple* and the reaction *slow*. It took hours for her suffering to begin.

Fortunately, we were able to single out the offending foods, and as long as Linda avoids them, she awakens refreshed in the morning.

Slow-developing food allergy presents further problems in diagnosis. It often perversely refuses to cooperate on the usual food skin tests, sometimes forcing us to abandon this highly useful tool. Other times the tests must be modified to search for delayed reactions (positive tests that take six to twenty-four hours to develop instead of the usual thirty minutes). These delayed tests can cause us to miss the diagnosis, and it is always hard to decide when to use them, or whether we need to modify the tests to accept, as positive, reactions different from the usual.

By now I think you have some understanding of the roadblocks we encounter in diagnosing the *slow-developing* and *multiple-food* allergies. You might think these are the last of the riddles we must solve as we unravel the mystery of a patient's food reactions. Unfortunately, you would be wrong; we haven't yet discussed the very important role of *accumulation* in concealing the foods that cause illness.

Accumulation

Most of us can identify with accumulation in the usual sense of the word. Remember that Thanksgiving dinner when you stuffed yourself until you felt like your stomach would burst? You just plain ate too much! You were horribly uncomfortable and berated yourself later for eating like a little piggy. You *accumulated* too much food and were unable to tolerate the sheer bulk in your tummy.

If you have food allergy, however, *accumulation* doesn't mean eating an amount of food so massive that your stomach is ready to burst. It means eating or drinking too much of the foods or beverages you *tolerate* poorly. Foods or beverages that won't hurt you in small quantities will bring pain and discomfort if you exceed that magic amount your body can handle.

With the quick-striking and dangerous food allergies, as well as with single-food allergies, and many times with multiple-food allergies, it takes only a small amount of food to bring illnesses. Patients can't tolerate any of the food. However, with accumulative food allergy, the patient *can* tolerate some of the food, but any quantity above this tolerance level and misfortune strikes.

This is frequently the case with food allergy. A lot of patients suffer if they exceed their tolerance level for certain foods and beverages—foods and beverages they *tolerate* poorly—and *accumulate* enough to bring on illness.

Although many quick-striking food reactions are dangerous and even deadly, these aren't. Slow-acting, accumulative food reactions cause pain and discomfort but usually aren't life threatening. And unlike quick-striking food reactions, which are usually easy to diagnose, accumulative reactions require a lot of detective work. Diagnosis can be frustrating and perplexing.

When our patients eat or drink too much of a food or beverage they tolerate poorly, a number of factors can conceal the cause of illness: multiple foods are usually involved; their effects can be additive; the time of onset of illness is variable; the foods are often considered healthy; they may be disguised by food craving; symptoms are usually multiple, with many ill-defined.

Earlier we discussed the difficulty of diagnosing food allergy when many foods are involved. This difficulty is compounded with accumulation when the effects of these foods are *additive*. Eating a small amount of a number of offending foods is the same as eating a large amount of one food. For instance, if too much orange juice makes your stomach cramp, you might think you can solve the problem by drinking only one little glass a day.

It's not that easy. If you don't realize that strawberries and tomatoes reinforce the painful effects of orange juice, your tummy will continue cramping and you will continue aching, discouraged because you feel you missed the diagnosis. Don't give up; there may be a family of foods bothering your stomach. Be glad you found one of them, and look for brother and sister foods that *add* to the distressing cramping caused by orange juice. Reducing those foods will probably calm your stomach.

How soon after a meal will symptoms strike? How long does it take to fill a bucket? The answers are the same. If the bucket is empty, it may take a long time to fill it. If it is full, it may slop over if you add a single drop of water. In accumulative food allergy, it may take hours to a day or more for illness to strike—or you may not even get sick—if you haven't had aggravating foods in your diet lately. You don't have enough in your body to cause a reaction. However, if enough of these foods were featured in your recent meals, you may be like that full bucket that can't hold even a tiny bit more water. You could react quickly. That's why the time from eating to onset of symptoms is *variable*. It can range from minutes to hours to days, a variation that can be very confusing to you and your doctor.

Time of onset also varies depending on the *amount consumed*. A little bit may be okay—no symptoms. A larger amount may cause a mild reaction the next day. A meal featuring lots of an aggravating food forces early and severe discomfort. Even more variability and more confusion.

I am reminded of Jack's case of migraine headaches. Jack owned a local franchise of a major restaurant chain, so his attention was naturally directed to foods as a possible cause for his migraines. But Jack was confused. Sometimes he was sure certain foods caused the migraines; the pain struck right after he ate them. Sometimes he was sure they didn't; he ate them without experiencing pain or the headache appeared the next day. When his neurologist couldn't explain these odd circumstances, he sent Jack to see me.

The answer was obvious. Jack was affected by **multiple** foods, his symptoms appeared only after he had **accumulated** enough to have a headache, the foods were **additive** in their effects, and all of this induced **variability** in the time of onset of his headache pain.

When we identified the group of foods that caused his migraines and explained why he experienced variability in his symptoms, Jack was able to avoid food-caused migraine headaches. As long as he doesn't cheat on his diet (he does at times), food doesn't give him headaches.

Two other factors interfere with the diagnosis of food allergy. One is craving. I don't know why the sublime architect of allergy ordained that many humans (not all) must crave the foods that harm them. Maybe it was that

rascal assistant architect who burdened us with this devil-
ish perversity. I do know that it often blocks a patient from
accepting our advice on which foods to avoid.

I know the craving factor is operating when a patient
tells me, "I can't believe these foods cause me any problems." Or, "That can't be right. These foods don't bother
me." These are characteristic responses from patients with
food cravings who don't even want to consider the possibility that the foods they love are causing their discomfort.
You might wonder how we can be so sure this is a form of
denial in certain patients. The answer is simple. After they
learn these foods really are bad for them—typically about
three years later—they admit their food cravings made
them reject our advice. (I don't know why it so often takes
three years, but it does.)

The other factor interfering with the diagnosis of food
allergy is past and present training. We are **conditioned** to
believe that certain foods are healthy; we are **persuaded**
that we must eat them every day because they are essential;
we are **convinced** that without them we are unhealthy.
Mama told us, teacher told us, and now dieticians and
other health experts tell us this is true. Unfortunately for
we allergic people, mama, teacher, and these other experts
were and are mistaken, but how hard it is for us to discard
this well-meant but wrong advice.

Each of the foods and food chemicals we will discuss in
this book are defended vociferously by acknowledged
experts in food science who honestly believe they are safe
and part of a healthy diet. Many scientific studies confirm
the conclusions of these experts. Unfortunately, the allergies of my patients deny the value and safety of these foods
for many allergic patients.

This lifelong conditioning is the reason so many allergic
folks continue to consume the foods and beverages that
harm them: "After all," they tell themselves, "orange juice
has a lot of vitamin C." It's also the reason so many doctors

are unaware of the illness certain foods can cause some allergic patients: "Can't be milk. It's such an important source of calcium." And it's also the reason a patient often resists our advice: "Can't be wheat. Mother always said bread was the staff of life."

Prior and present conditioning definitely complicate the diagnosis and treatment of food allergy. So many people find it ridiculous to even suspect that the vitamin-packed glass of orange juice clutched in their fists also packs a lot of misery. Persuading them otherwise is often quite a job.

It's Not Hopeless

This lengthy discussion of the complexity of food allergy might suggest that diagnosis is hopeless, but that's not really the case. It is true that sometimes we fail to diagnose or help our food-sensitive patients, but in most cases we succeed because food allergy has one helpful trait. Each food (or group of foods) tends to cause characteristic symptoms. Not all the time, but enough times to be helpful in diagnosis. After years of diagnosing and treating food allergy, a doctor is able to recognize and use this tendency to help his patients.

Another factor that makes the diagnosis and treatment of food allergy possible is that certain foods, beverages, and food chemicals are almost always the worst offenders. They share the characteristics we already discussed: they are *multiple, accumulative, additive,* and they cause symptoms that are *variable in time of onset.* Once a patient recognizes and determines his or her *tolerance* for them, a lot of the mystery surrounding food allergy disappears. These extremely important foods and beverages are the focus of this book.

Citrus

The events that change our thinking are often peculiar. They usually leave a lasting impression because they are so strange and surprising. They challenge our deeply held beliefs, our concept of order, our most sacred convictions. They turn our view of the world upside down—and stick in our memories.

I remember just such an event, the event that forced me to develop a food allergy diet.

A Peculiar Event

It was 1965, and I was a captain in the U.S. Air Force, stationed at Offutt Air Force Base in Omaha, Nebraska. Medical school and internship completed, I was serving as a GMO (General Medical Officer) at the base hospital and clinic. There were a number of clinics, including pediatrics, internal medicine, OB-GYN, and several other specialty clinics, but there was no allergy clinic because, before I arrived on base, no doctor had been interested in this specialty. Well, I was interested. Even though I had no allergy training at that time, I realized we could improve the care of the allergic patients on base if we had a clinic that combined a doctor interested in allergy with nurses trained in allergy. I decided to start an allergy clinic.

One of my first allergy patients was five-year-old Susie, dark-haired and adorable, a little sprite with the behavior of a scamp—and skin the texture of course-grained sandpaper. She was suffering from a horrible case of eczema. Her skin was dry, thick, and red, and her constant itching and scratching made her days and nights miserable. Although this aggravating affliction didn't seem to dim her sunny disposition, I felt so sorry for her. I could see this same pity in the eyes of her father Bob, who brought her repeatedly to my clinic hoping I could help.

I tried. I prescribed all the treatments that are supposed to relieve eczema symptoms—antihistamines, salves, lotions, avoiding soap, cutting fingernails short, and wearing gloves at night to reduce damage caused by scratching. The results were frustratingly inadequate.

Then, one day Bob brought Susie in and she looked great! There had to be a seventy-five percent improvement in the condition of her skin, and she was no longer red as a lobster.

"Bob, Susie looks great." I said.

"She sure does," he replied.

"I was hoping my treatment would do Susie some good, Bob, and it looks like it finally did," I said, my head swelling with pride that I had been able to conquer Susie's severe eczema, grateful that my training and knowledge could provide such excellent results.

"Well . . . , not exactly," said Bob, with an odd look on his face.

"What do you mean, 'not exactly'?" I asked

"Well," said Bob, "none of those things helped Susie very much. She has her own way of treatment."

"Her own treatment? What is it?" I asked, wondering what it could possibly be.

"Well, when her skin gets really bad, she dumps kitchen cleanser into a bathtub full of water and jumps in. Clears her skin right up."

I was so astonished by his answer you could have knocked me over with a feather. In fact, I would have dropped if someone had waved a feather anywhere in the vicinity. Such humbling experiences are typical in my life. It seems like whenever I start thinking how smart I am, something happens to deflate my ego, letting me know I still have a lot to learn. All my fancy treatments were no match for Susie's. Move over, you gods of medical progress— Madame Curie with your x-ray machine and Alexander Fleming with your discovery of penicillin—here comes Susie with her kitchen cleanser!

Before we go any further, I want you to understand that I am not advocating your self-treatment of eczema with a bath of kitchen cleanser. I have no idea whether kitchen cleanser baths are harmful, so please don't try them.

I wasn't sure what lesson I was to learn from Susie. It was like listening to the beating of distant drums; I could sense there was a message in it for me, but I didn't know how long it would be before I could understand it. What I did know was that I wanted to help children and adults with eczema, to come up with treatments that would have better results than those available at the time provided. And I somehow knew that before I could unlock the mystery surrounding the diagnosis and treatment of eczema, I would need specialty training in allergy and the practical knowledge I would accumulate over years of treating allergic patients.

Another Peculiar Event

Before I could begin to grasp the point of Susie's lesson, however, another peculiar event occurred, one that was no less surprising than the first. Like my experience with

Susie, it made me doubt things I firmly believed to be true, made me discard tried and true methods, and shook the very foundations of everything I had been taught about allergy.

It happened years later, after I finished allergy specialty training at the Mayo Clinic and started my practice in St. Paul. It was the fall of 1973, my third year of practice, and increasing numbers of patients were visiting my office. One of these patients was a seven-year-old boy named Mike, a bright boy with the solemn manner of a supreme court judge and skin that was dry, scaly, and inflamed. In retrospect, his skin was a lot like Susie's, although it didn't occur to me at the time. If it had, perhaps I might have been prepared for the surprise that awaited me in Mike's case.

Treatment of eczema hadn't improved much since I had had Susie as a patient; results were still frustratingly inadequate. Mike had been sent to me by his dermatologist to see if I could find any causes for his rash. I wasn't too hopeful, since medical science still didn't understand eczema very well.

Mike, his mother Karen, and I tried various eczema treatments for several months without making any progress; Mike was as red and itchy as the day he first came to my office. Then, on one of Mike's visits, Karen and I had a conversation that forever changed my thinking on and treatment of eczema. I still remember that day.

"Well, Karen, how's Mike doing?" I asked.

"No change, Doctor Walsh. He's still uncomfortable and itches as much as always."

"That's too bad, Karen. I wish we could be more effective in treating him, but it's hard to do much when we don't even know the cause of eczema." Then I asked, "Karen, have you noticed anything that makes his eczema worse?"

Karen didn't take long to answer. "Yes, I have," she said. "His skin flares up whenever he eats or drinks too much citrus."

Her answer stunned me. Karen had always impressed me as being a practical and bright woman, not at all likely to be led astray by those old folk tales that blame the acids in foods for imagined illnesses. Allergy experts I respected discredited such addled-brained theories, maintaining that they were the invention of the charlatan doctor and the neurotic patient. It couldn't be true, and of that I was sure! Being relatively new to practice, I still hadn't learned to trust my patient, and I still had the inflated ego of the newly trained specialist—I fought against any new ideas that contradicted the teachings I had so laboriously pounded into my head. Thankfully, the realities of medical practice eventually deflate that ego.

Karen's belief that citrus caused Mike's eczema was contrary to everything I knew about allergy. Most allergists agree that eczema is strongly stimulated by allergy, but the idea that patients could be allergic to citrus was preposterous.

Karen's conclusion didn't make sense for a couple of reasons. First, although people who are allergic to such things as seafood or ragweed react to only tiny parts of the food or pollen, the parts must be at least a certain size. If they are too small, there is no allergic reaction. Citrus is too small. Like the toy poodle at the dog track, it doesn't belong in the race at all.

Second, most of the allergies we know about are directed against proteins; citrus isn't a protein. Most allergies are directed against proteins foreign to the body; citrus isn't foreign. In fact, *citric acid* is present in every cell in the body and is one of the compounds involved in energy production. Again, this toy poodle didn't belong in the race.

"Karen, you surprise me," I said. "I thought the fear of food acids was dead and buried. What makes you think citrus bothers Mike?"

"Because he breaks out badly if he eats oranges or grapefruit," she answered, "and he is also miserable if he drinks citrus juices or pop flavored with citrus."

I still wasn't convinced, but I put aside my skepticism for the moment and said, "Okay. Let's get citrus out of his diet and see what happens." I figured it couldn't hurt; I wasn't helping Mike much anyway.

Over the next several weeks, Karen eliminated from Mike's diet all citrus fruits, their juices, and any beverages flavored with citric acid such as pop and sports drinks. Mike's skin improved remarkably. And not only did his skin improve with citrus eliminated, returning these foods and beverages to his diet made his skin red, scaly, and itchy again. Karen was right; it was citrus—the toy poodle of allergy—that was making Mike miserable.

The results made me glad I had overcome my skepticism, and once I absorbed the implications of citrus-caused allergy, I was eager to try citrus elimination on patients with other allergic illnesses. I tried it on patients with abdominal cramps and diarrhea; the cramps diminished and the diarrhea subsided. I tried it on patients with hives; the hives were less severe. I tried it on patients with stuffed noses; the stuffiness decreased. Asthmatic patients wheezed less. Even hay fever patients responded to elimination; if they avoided citrus their pollen reactions eased up. I was impressed and excited.

Obviously citrus bothered a lot of my patients and was important in many of their allergic illnesses. But why? I can't say for sure, but I suspect it may have something to do with the human body's ability to adapt to change. Even though each one of our cells contains a small amount of citric acid, our bodies may be unable to handle large amounts of food acids. This is probably because these large quantities of acidic foods are a recent addition to our diets, and our digestive, metabolic, and elimination processes haven't yet adjusted to dealing with them.

I know this may seem surprising, since experts believe citrus cultivation started in China *four thousand years ago*. But when you consider that we digest, metabolize, and eliminate our food the same way as those primitive homo sapiens who first dodged the footsteps of dinosaurs *eighty million years ago*, four thousand years is but a blink of evolution's eye. Not enough time to *evolve* an innovative ability to handle a *new* diet.

Our modern food production system is partly responsible for us consuming huge amounts of food acids—just check the ingredients on the canned and packaged foods in your pantry to see how many contain acidic ingredients. And our present generation's eating habits have increased the incidence of acidic foods in our diet—*grapefruit juice* in the morning, *tomato* slices in our sandwiches and an *orange* at noon, *potatoes* and *strawberry* ice cream at dinner, and *grapes* as a late-night snack.

This list emphasizes another surprising point; all of the foods mentioned are acidic. I didn't know foods such as strawberries and potatoes were acidic when Karen told me about Mike's reaction to citric acid, but I learned they were when I learned about certain inconsistencies that arose in treating other patients. Why did Dick's migraines strike when he drank apple juice, which contains mostly *malic acid*? Why did Alice's diarrhea flare up after eating candy with *fumaric acid*? Obviously, allergic distress was being caused by acids other then citric acid.

Citric, fumaric, malic acids—the names are familiar. Each of them participates in the Krebs cycle, the process that changes food to energy. As energy is released, the acids are torn apart, changing them from one acid into another. Citric acid changes to succinic acid, succinic acid to fumaric, fumaric to malic, then—after a little repair to the torn-up acid—back to citric acid again.

Of all the acids we find in our diet, citric acid is most important because it is the one most widely used. Its pleasant, sour, fruity taste makes it a perfect flavoring agent for beverages, candy, pies, and many other treats. It is often used in the pharmaceutical industry, usually in amounts too small to cause symptoms. Except in one case I remember well.

I met Jean, a seventy-six-year-old retired kindergarten teacher, when her internist asked me to examine her in the hospital just after her bowel surgery. Prior to surgery, she was given medicine to clear all the stool out of her colon. The medicine worked too well—she had a frightful case of diarrhea. Not only did she have diarrhea, she had such hypotension she almost went into shock, and it took days for her to recover from this overpowering reaction. Her internist and surgeon were stumped: "All we gave her was a dose of harmless magnesium citrate," they told me. *Citrate* is another name for citrus, and after battling my patient's citrus-caused diarrhea, I wasn't stumped by what happened at all, nor did I think citrate was harmless. However, the experience did help me realize that other doctors had no concept of the illness that could be caused in certain allergic patients by large doses of citrus.

Malic acid, the major acid in apples, is second in importance and frequency of use to citric acid. Much like citric acid, it has a pleasant, sour, fruity taste and is used to flavor foods and beverages and in pharmaceutical products.

Fumaric and succinic acids are seldom used in foods or beverages, although I have noticed fumaric in some candies, and both are used in drug manufacturing, where the levels seem too low to bother my patients. The names of these acids can sometimes be confusing. For all practical purposes, citrate and citric acid are the same, as are succinate and succinic acid, fumarate and fumaric acid, and malate and malic acid.

The more I investigate acidic foods and their effect on my poor patients, the more complicated it becomes. Multiple foods, multiple illnesses, multiple acids. Every time I think I finally understand it all, new information surfaces. It's like carrying a sheet of four-by-eight foot plywood on a windy day—every time you take four steps forward, a new gust comes along and blows you two steps backward.

For instance, just as I was congratulating myself on knowing all the acids that made my patients sick, I found a new one. *Tartaric acid* or tartrate, the main acid in grapes, grape juice, grape-flavored drinks, wine, and brandy, causes particularly severe reactions in my patients, illnesses such as headaches, hives, eczema, cramps, diarrhea and many others. That discovery taught me to be constantly on the lookout, and even now, although the diet works well for my patients, I am sure I haven't identified all the foods, illnesses, or acids that may cause problems. In treating food allergy, keeping an open mind is essential.

When I first began telling my patients they might be allergic to acidic foods, they were overwhelmed by the complexity of changing their eating habits, and I couldn't blame them for looking at me with evident confusion and asking, "What should I avoid?" A mumbled response that they should avoid all acidic foods didn't ease their confusion one bit. They needed to have the diet written down so they could understand it, so I began to do so. And revised it when my staff and I learned more. And revised it again and again and again. And that's how the diet has evolved to where it is today.

I believe that understanding the role of acidic foods is a significant advance in the science of medicine and the diagnosis and treatment of medical illness. But lest you think I am praising myself, let me hasten to say I didn't discover it. Susie and her kitchen cleanser baths, Karen and her theory on citrus, as well as many other patients who contributed their insights—they all helped.

By the way, I'm sure you must be wondering why it helped when Susie bathed with kitchen cleanser. I have to confess I'm not sure, but I think I know. Susie was neutralizing the acidity of her skin by soaking in bath water turned basic by kitchen cleanser. It is a basic law of chemistry that in solution, bases neutralize acids. I believe that in cases like Susie's, the body is trying to eliminate the excess acid in the diet by dumping it on the skin, where it causes the redness, scaliness, and obnoxious itching characteristic of eczema.

Perhaps Susie's kitchen cleanser is a key to learning the cause of this annoying condition.

Monosodium Glutamate (Alias MSG)

A doctor's mission and calling is to nurture, protect, and improve his patients' precious health. This honorable mission imposes a heavy burden of responsibility on members of the medical profession, an obligation to shield our patients and the community at large against what we perceive as dangerous. I believe all doctors feel this obligation. I know I do.

For me, nothing heightens this sense of obligation more than monosodium glutamate, a food chemical my staff and I try our darnedest to eliminate from our patients' diets. I don't mean to be an alarmist, but I am deeply worried by the frequency with which I encounter its effects in my practice and its presence in so much of what we eat. Perhaps when I tell you about some of my experiences with this dietary chemical, you'll understand my concern.

Citrus Wasn't Enough

I was delighted with the improvement in my patient's symptoms when the significance of the acidic foods and beverages became apparent. When patients reduced or

41

eliminated them, headaches decreased, cramps and diarrhea slowed down, hives sprouted less often, eczema itched less, noses unblocked, and wheezing declined.

However, I was also perplexed. Although my patient's symptoms diminished, they did not disappear. In fact they still had plenty of headaches, hives, diarrhea, and all the other maladies to which the allergic person is prey. I had to improve the diet.

Fortunately, I was able to find a number of good references that helped. Through them I learned that many foods other then oranges, lemons, limes, and grapefruit are acidic. Tomatoes, berries, and cherries are acidic, often more so than the citrus fruits. And the acid in grapes—tartaric acid—can stimulate especially vicious allergic symptoms. Apparently, that's why so many of my patients can't drink wine.

That the ordinary potato is acid came as quite a shock to me. It wasn't even on my list of suspects. The potato seems to be related to the tomato; to me the leaves look like tomato leaves and the seed looks like a tiny green tomato. That helps explain why many of my patients suffer if they eat potatoes. I found that potatoes cause the same symptoms as tomatoes if eaten in excess of my patient's tolerance level, a level that is sometimes very low.

Each new finding was added to the diet, each new finding helped my patients, but I was still puzzled. Although there were pleasing improvements, my patients still had plenty of symptoms. Why? What was missing?

What was missing was my willingness to listen to my patients. I hadn't yet learned the lesson that the ones who knows the most about the course of my patients' illnesses and the environmental factors that are affecting them are the patients themselves. They were telling me about other ingredients in the diet that made them ill, foods that were not acidic. I was finally forced into recognizing this by a friend who suffered with cluster headaches.

Another Ingredient in the Diet

Although the many allergies bestowed on me include sinus headache, I am fortunate in never having experienced cluster headaches, one of the most painful of human afflictions. In cluster headaches, the nerves of the face and scalp ache with overwhelming intensity. John had such headaches and had tried every medical treatment known. His only relief was to inhale pure oxygen when one of these painful headaches struck.

I tried treating him with allergy injections and eliminating acid from his diet. It helped, but he still had unexplained headaches. Then one day John complained of a particularly brutal headache, which prompted the following discussion.

"Bill, I had a horrible headache last night."

"How did it happen, John?" I asked.

"I was at a meeting where they served snacks," he said. "I wasn't hungry, but you know how you munch just to keep your hands busy. I ate some sausages that were excellent. On the way home I got hit with a headache so painful I had trouble seeing where I was driving. It was so bad I wasn't able to break it with oxygen," he sighed. "The pain kept me up all night."

"John, did you eat anything else?" I wondered.

"No."

"Did you drink anything?" I tried again.

"Just water," he replied, shrugging his shoulders.

I felt sorry for John. He looked pale and worn out after his night of dreadful pain. I was also curious—was there some clue to John's pain in that sausage? We tracked down the ingredients and found that they included monosodium glutamate.

I remembered that patients had often told me monosodium glutamate (also known as MSG) caused them headaches or diarrhea, but I had dismissed their observations, theorizing that it wasn't the MSG but their own imagination that was at fault. After all, studies by medical scientists showed that monosodium glutamate rarely, if ever, caused illness. But I was to find my patients observations were right.

What Is Monosodium Glutamate?

For those who aren't familiar with MSG aside from seeing it listed among those strange-sounding, synthetic chemicals on food product labels, a short description might be useful. First of all, it's not strange or unnatural; it's found in your body proteins. And it's also not synthetic. Every plant and animal manufactures it.

Proteins are made of individual amino acids, much as a chain is made of individual links. Glutamic acid is one of the amino acid links in protein, where it makes up from ten to forty percent of various proteins (that's a lot). When glutamic acid is freed from the protein chain, it is soluble (floats) in water or body fluids, where it meets a sodium molecule (part of table salt) that floats with it. Hence the name monosodium (one salt) glutamate (free glutamic acid)—shortened to MSG. (Sodium glutamate would be an adequate name, but someone must have decided monosodium glutamate sounded classier.)

How does it harm my patients? I believe the problem does not stem from the glutamic acid in protein, where it is bound firmly and released slowly, slowly enough so the body can handle it at its own pace. Free glutamic acid, MSG, is not bound to protein and is probably absorbed so fast that the body's metabolism is overwhelmed. It can't handle it. Foods and beverages with high levels of MSG make my patients sick with dependable regularity.

Illness Caused by MSG

The illness caused by MSG varies among patients. Debbie, a thirty-one-year-old labor and delivery nurse from one of our local hospitals, recently told me about her reactions.

"How are the allergy shots treating you, Debbie?"

"They help a lot as long as I get them every two weeks," she said. "If I let them go beyond two weeks, my nose gets stuffy and I feel tired."

"How about your diet? Any foods give you trouble?" I asked.

"I have to avoid the acid foods or my cold sores flare up. As a nurse I look horrible with a big cold sore on my lips, and my patients think I have some terrible disease."

"Any trouble with MSG, Debbie?"

"I have to avoid it completely. I read every label, so it's not too hard to avoid in my own cooking, but sometimes I'll eat it at a restaurant or at dinner at a friend's house. I'm too embarrassed to ask them if they use MSG," she admitted. They'd probably think I'm a kook."

"I know what you mean about eating at a friend's house," I sympathized. "What does MSG do to you?"

"It's really bad, Doctor Walsh. First of all I develop a terrible thirst. Then I get puffy and bloated and my clothes get real tight, and I can't wear a belt because my stomach hurts. I get hyper, and for several nights I can't sleep. And all my joints ache."

Debbie's reaction to MSG is not rare, unusual, or a figment of her imagination. Many other patients complain of these symptoms, and I also share them. I always ask at a restaurant if they use MSG and try to choose foods that aren't likely to contain it, but sometimes I get it anyway. My good friends know not to use it in meals they prepare for me, but I feel strange questioning the hostess about MSG if I don't know her well. Like Debbie, I don't want to sound like a kook.

When I get MSG, it gets me. Hours later a huge thirst develops; I feel puffy and bloated—my hands swell so much they feel like sausages. My belt hurts and my bathroom scale creeps upward, showing five extra pounds that stay for about three days, then drop off. (I often wonder how many people who are taking "water pills" for fluid accumulation share this problem.) After eating foods with MSG, I sleep miserably for about three nights until the bloating stops and the scale drops. My stomach churns with acid, and like Debbie, I have nagging joint pain; my bad knee swells and aches for three days.

So for many patients MSG causes puffiness, bloating, abdominal discomfort, joint achiness, irritability, and insomnia. And the list of symptoms goes on and on. For others, their asthma worsens, their noses stuff and their ears block, hives flare, and eczema itches more. For those who react with headaches, their sinus pressure increases measurably, and migraine sufferers experience nearly unbearable surges of pain. (I don't think any of my numerous patients with frequent headaches can tolerate MSG.)

In the majority of my patients who develop pain and discomfort from MSG, although the reactions brought on by this food additive are not life-threatening, they find its effects so devastating that many must avoid it as they would avoid playing with a loaded gun.

At the same time, the subject of MSG must be approached with a sense of proportion. It does not cause all allergic symptoms, although it causes many. Allergy is too complex a matter to attribute all symptoms to a single food or food chemical; logic tells us there have to be multiple causes for these numerous illnesses. However, it is important to recognize that, in my patients, this dietary component often provokes uncomfortable, painful, and even dangerous illness. I suspect that my patients are not atypical and that many other allergic people share this susceptibility to MSG.

Where Is MSG Found?

When I began looking for acidic foods, I foolishly thought they would be easy to find. Instead, I found there were many sources and types of acids, and they could crop up in the strangest places. It was the same with MSG.

At first I thought, *What could be easier?* Read your labels, stop using spices that contain MSG, and when you dine out, tell the waitress you want your meal prepared without MSG. The problem is solved. Unfortunately, it's not that easy.

When you tell the waitress not to use MSG, she often looks at you with a confused expression and asks, "What's MSG?" Or, even worse, she will attempt to appease you by assuring you, "We don't use MSG in our cooking," and then unwittingly brings you a meal loaded with it. How often that's happened to me.

Reading labels is the right thing to do, but you *must read every label.* MSG is used to enhance the flavor of many dishes, especially meat, breading, and soups, but you can find it anywhere in the diet. Read every label, *always.*

MSG must be mentioned on every label where it is used in its pure form. However, if a food processor added it as hydrolyzed vegetable protein, it can be present in a food without being listed on the label. It's a sneaky and underhanded way to do it and often catches my patients by surprise.

Hydrolyzed vegetable protein is simply vegetable protein that is hydrolyzed or broken down into amino acids. Since protein, including vegetable protein, is ten to forty percent glutamic acid, hydrolyzed vegetable protein contains between *ten and forty percent monosodium glutamate.* (Remember, protein-bound glutamic acid doesn't hurt my patients. The harm comes when the glutamic acid is released from the protein and becomes the free and rapidly absorbed monosodium glutamate.)

I once went to a food show where soup processors were proudly advertising their "MSG-free" products. When I read the label, I noticed that each soup contained hydrolyzed vegetable protein. I'm afraid I made a spectacle of myself berating the poor salespeople about their suspicious advertising practices and telling them that if my patients ate their soups, they would become exceedingly ill. I didn't make any headway, but you can make a difference if you see a product with hydrolyzed vegetable protein that is not labeled as containing MSG. Complain to the store manager—he doesn't want to lose you as a customer. When *he* complains to the food companies, perhaps they will listen and admit to using MSG in their product.

By the way, when dining in a restaurant, ask for a simple meat, fish, or poultry dish—no sauces—and ask that no spices of any sort be put on it. Then hope for the best.

Fermentation and MSG

I thought I had discovered all the sources of MSG when I found it in spices and in hydrolyzed vegetable protein. I was wrong. Some of my patients told me they had MSG-like symptoms when they ate cheese. That sounded strange because cheese is made of milk, and milk doesn't have high levels of MSG, but I searched and found reference books on MSG which explained the mystery. (Actually, I should have figured this one out myself.)

Milk protein is twenty percent glutamic acid, most of it firmly bound to protein so that the body can slowly digest and absorb it. However, in the cheese-making process, the milk protein is fermented, breaking apart the protein and releasing MSG. It seems that the more aged the cheese, the more MSG it contains. In fact, much to my distress, as I like cheese, some of the foods highest in MSG are varieties of aged cheese. What a shame.

Any fermentation process will break down protein, releasing MSG. Soy sauce is a frequently used fermentation product, and my patients find they must avoid it or suffer severe consequences. Fermentation may also be one of the reasons so many allergic patients can't tolerate alcoholic drinks. Most of my food-sensitive patients react severely to wine, probably because the combination of citric and tartaric acids plus the fermentation-released MSG is devastating. The moral of the story? Beware of all fermented preparations.

Before leaving the subject of fermentation, I should mention autolyzed yeast extract. Yeast extract has the ability to autolyze or break down its own protein, releasing MSG. Avoid foods with autolyzed yeast extract.

High Free Glutamate Levels in Certain Foods

Another discovery I have made in reading about this problem is that certain foods naturally contain high levels of free glutamic acid or MSG, and patients with sensitivity to MSG must approach them cautiously. They include peas, corn, mushrooms, and tomatoes.

Eating *peas* and *corn* may be acceptable for many MSG-sensitive people. I suspect a good boiling will remove much of the water-soluble MSG, especially in corn when it is removed from the cob before boiling. Cutting it from the cob also cuts each kernel, exposing it to the boiling water.

I have personal experience with corn intolerance. I consider corn on the cob to be one of the foods of the gods. I love its sweet, succulent taste, especially when drenched in butter, but it doesn't love me. Corn on the cob gives me all the same symptoms I get from eating MSG—bloating, acid stomach, insomnia—but corn cut from the cob and then boiled is okay. A surprising number of my patients share similar experiences.

Mushrooms and *tomatoes* cannot be processed the same way. In fact, removing the MSG from these foods would probably make them so bland we wouldn't care to have them in our diet. The combination of MSG and acid in tomatoes must be the reason they are so highly prized as flavoring in our foods. The presence of both must also be the reason my patients complain so bitterly of their effects. Watch out for peas, corn, mushrooms, and tomatoes!

Overriding Concerns

The impact of MSG on my patients is enormous; it causes severe illness. Its constant presence in our diet makes it difficult to avoid, but the misery it causes my patients makes avoidance imperative. It is hard for me to believe my patients are the only allergic people affected by MSG. The odds are that many more people are susceptible, and I am concerned that they are unaware of it. Being unaware, they have no way of knowing they should avoid this chemical.

I also worry that MSG may be causing more harm than the allergic illness I see in my practice. There is good evidence MSG is *neurotoxic*; that is, it damages nerves. The implications of this neurotoxicity are profound, and we will examine them as we discuss other dietary chemicals that my patients must avoid.

Low-Calorie Sweeteners

Of all the dietary chemicals we ask our patients to avoid, I have the least experience with low-calorie food and beverage sweeteners.

This is not the case with other dietary chemicals. Patients respond favorably when we advise them to eliminate MSG and really try to abstain from its use, but it is hard to escape this omnipresent chemical. It is added to many foods and spices as MSG or hydrolyzed vegetable protein. Fermentation releases it from milk (cheese), soy (soy sauce), various grains, and grapes (alcoholic beverages). It is even present naturally in foods such as mushrooms and corn. Our patients find it almost impossible to consistently avoid the excess quantities that make them ill.

Avoiding acidic food is also hard; the sources are so numerous and acidic foods and beverages so delicious.

Because my patients happen onto MSG-laced meals or devour too much acidic food on many occasions, not a day goes by when I don't hear at least one or two stories of pain and suffering from their use. These stories keep problems caused by acidic foods and MSG fresh in my mind.

Not so with low-calorie sweeteners. They are easy to identify, and our patients seem to have an innate suspicion of them. Most patients eliminate them from their diet immediately and never return to using them. Therefore, it is harder to define the symptoms they stimulate.

My best glimpse at these symptoms comes when new patients who have been using high quantities of low-calorie sweeteners stop their use, or with those few patients who continue using them while following the rest of our dietary advice. These chemicals seems to cause the same symptoms we see with MSG—headache, bloating, irritability, hives, eczema, abdominal cramps, diarrhea, nasal blockage, wheezing, joint and muscle aches, plus many others—and eliminating them seems to reverse those symptoms.

Although I have less experience with low-calorie sweeteners than with other components of the diet, I believe they cause illnesses and I also believe my patients must avoid them. Proceeding on the assumption that this is correct, let's examine them further.

What are the Low-Calorie Sweeteners?

The two most widely used sweeteners are saccharin and aspartame. Saccharin is not frequently used by my patients; however, a number of them use aspartame, which sweetens a multitude of foods and beverages, including breakfast cereal, chewing gum, cocoa, instant iced tea, and alcoholic beverage mixes. Equal®, a granulated sugar substitute, is made of aspartame. NutraSweet®—aspartame again— sweetens many carbonated and noncarbonated beverages.

Aspartame is made of aspartic acid and phenylalanine, two of the twenty or so amino acids that the body uses to make protein. (We already know that MSG or glutamic acid is another of these amino acids.) Although they are bound together in the aspartame molecule, this molecule seems to break apart rapidly in digestion, releasing both amino acids and allowing rapid absorption into the body (as in the case of MSG).

The phenylalanine component of aspartame raises some concern. Phenylalanine causes brain damage in infants with a medical disorder called phenylketonuria, which affects about one in twelve thousand white and Asian babies and a lower percentage of African-American babies. Two percent of us carry one of the two genes necessary to pass this disorder to our children. Infants with phenylketonuria become profoundly retarded if dietary phenylalanine is not rigidly limited.

Obviously those who have this disorder should be avoiding aspartame, and it seems to me that anyone who uses this chemical frequently should be asking: Will long-term dietary use of phenylalanine eventually harm even those who do not have phenylketonuria? Although this would be an interesting concept to dwell on, we won't. We are more concerned with the aspartic acid component of aspartame.

Aspartic Acid

I knew about aspartic acid, but I didn't pay much attention to it until it was mentioned in some material I was reading about the glutamic acid element of MSG. I was fortunate in finding a number of reference books on glutamic acid, as well as symposium papers and textbooks written by scientists who are studying it. I was unfortunate in not being able to thoroughly understand what they were saying. Most of the papers were directed at scientists who are familiar with the jargon of the field and not at the occasional allergist who might try to read them. (Allergists have their own jargon, but I've tried to spare you many of the incomprehensible words we use.)

Even though I did not fully comprehend those references, I understood certain facts that pointed to an explanation of my patients' unfortunate reactions to the dietary chemicals we ask them to avoid. Although the following is speculative, I believe it is true. I also believe you deserve to know these facts. They explain *why* these chemicals must be avoided.

Excitotoxic Amino Acids

In the reference works I studied, aspartic acid and glutamic acid (MSG) were mentioned together because their actions are similar. Both are able to *excite* or stimulate nerve cells of animals, including humans. In excess quantities, especially in the young animal, both are *neurotoxic,* or poisonous to nerves. They are excitotoxic amino acids that can cause nerve degeneration. That's worrisome!

Of course, our ordinary diet does not subject us to the excessive quantity of these amino acids that caused nerve damage in the animal experiments. But what if there were a population of humans that suffered nerve degeneration from *long-term, low-dose exposure* in the diet? Perhaps the threat would be even greater if other diet chemicals, such as food acids, *potentiated* or aided in this damage. What if we called this population of people *allergic patients*?

Evidence

I know this theory probably sounds a little preposterous, but there is a great deal of evidence to support it. The following are examples of allergic illnesses in which nerve degeneration is a factor.

Cold sores, those recurring and unattractive ulcers of the lips, are caused by a virus infection of the nerves of the lips. My patients find that if they closely follow our dietary recommendations, especially if they drastically reduce their intake of acidic foods, their cold sores remain tiny and almost unnoticeable. In fact, I know this first hand because I get cold sores myself. Dietary avoidance does not cure cold sores, but it stops the spread of the lip rash. Evidently, the chemicals in foods (especially acids) further injure the virus-damaged nerve that is causing the ulcer, indicating they are neurotoxic to that nerve.

Another piece of evidence that is particularly impressive is found in eczema, the irritating skin disease that is marked by constant severe itching. Biopsies of eczema skin show badly damaged nerves. Many regard this evidence of *nerve degeneration* to be a consequence of eczema, but what if it is actually the cause? The answer, of course, is to remove any neurotoxic chemicals from the diet. By now, you shouldn't be surprised when I tell you that removing acidic foods, MSG, and aspartic acid from the diet almost always reduces the itchiness, allowing my patients to improve markedly.

I could give you many more examples of allergic illnesses, including such common afflictions as headaches, asthma, and hives, that give evidence of nerve degeneration or excitation. In each case, the evidence is intriguing and, I'd like to think, persuasive. Suffice it to say that these examples support my theory that dietary chemicals, including food acids, may contribute to nerve damage.

This theory is especially significant because it is *key* to explaining a great deal about food allergy. It helps in understanding *why* certain things happen. For instance, why does food allergy affect so many areas of the body? It also helps explain *how* these food chemicals cause unrelated illnesses such as diarrhea and hives in the same patient.

Relationship Between Allergic Symptoms

It might not seem like allergic symptoms that affect different areas of the body are related, but they are. Food chemicals do not need to attack the colon and skin directly, just the nerves supplying the colon and the skin. The irritated nerves throw the colon into spasm, causing abdominal pain and diarrhea. In the skin, this same damage will fire off the motor nerves, dilating blood vessels (making the skin red) and allowing fluid to leak from these dilated vessels (causing the hive bump). The damaged sensory nerves in the dilated blood vessels send itch sensations to the brain. That's why we often see abdominal pain and diarrhea as well as red, itchy, bumpy skin as part of the same allergic reaction.

Nerve damage caused by dietary chemicals can also explain other allergic illnesses. In migraine headaches, the damaged nerves controlling the blood vessels of the head dilate these vessels, stretching the surrounding nerve fibers. These stretched nerve fibers ache with each pulse of blood flowing through the blood vessels, resulting in the throbbing pain associated with migraine headache.

In patients with asthma, irritated nerves controlling the air passages fire off signals that constrict the muscles of the airway and swell the lining. Airflow to the lungs decreases and my patient wheezes. In patients with nasal stuffiness, irritated and damaged nerves swell the lining of the nasal passages, blocking the nose.

We could continue to examine the role of nerve damage in numerous other allergic illnesses, but I think the examples discussed show how all these diverse illness can share the same cause—*nerve irritation and damage caused by neuroexcitatory and neurotoxic food chemicals.*

How Does This Damage Occur?

I do not know for sure, but it intrigues me that all these food chemicals—the various food acids, MSG, and aspartic acid—are prominent in the Krebs cycle. In this important process, acids are torn apart in steps, each step changing one acid to another while producing energy, the basic energy that "powers up" each cell in our bodies.

Energy production is an enormously complicated process requiring many separate subprocesses to make it work. In the allergic person, one or more of these subprocesses must be faulty or marginal, unable to tolerate any disruption. The sudden flooding of the digestive process by the various food acids or the exitotoxic amino acids is most likely the cause of that disruption.

How are nerves injured? Nerves have special metabolic needs that may be especially vulnerable to the flooding that occurs during the Krebs cycle. Excess accumulation of aspartic, glutamic, or food acids may be particularly injurious in the allergic patient.

Different Strokes for Different Folks

Different patients exhibit different symptoms when they eat and drink the chemicals we ask them to avoid. Some experience diarrhea, some have headaches, some get hives, while still others suffer from wheezing or stuffy noses. Why do allergic people show such variation in symptoms? I believe genetics and injury account for the difference.

In our practice, we treat many families with several allergy-prone members, and I am amazed by the similarity in symptoms within each family. In some, painful migraine headaches are common to many members. In other families, headaches are as rare as a Minnesota summer without mosquitos, but eczema affects both parents and children. Some gene or combination of genes dictates a weakness for headaches or eczema. In other words, I think these patients have a *genetic predisposition* for certain illnesses.

I am convinced that *injury* is another major reason patients' symptoms appear where they do. Many of our food-sensitive patients experience severe headache pain that begins in an area of the neck that has been injured by whiplash. Those with arthritis experience painful aching in the joints when they ignore their diet. Patients with intestinal inflammatory diseases such as chronic ulcerative colitis find that dietary chemicals stimulate their abdominal distress.

Injury caused by accident or disease often dictates where allergic illness will strike. Whiplash, arthritis, and inflammatory bowel disease are not *caused* by allergy, but they are *aggravated* by it. Allergy is a despicable bully because it is attracted to areas of injury, where it intensifies the pain and discomfort that already exist. That explains why many patients with illnesses which are not caused by allergy are so frequently helped by allergy treatment. It is the cop that chases away the bully.

Aspartic Acid in the Diet

Fortunately, aspartic acid is encountered less frequently in our diet than acidic foods and MSG. As with MSG, we are not concerned with the aspartic acid that is locked into protein. Digestion is slowed by the need to break the amino acid free of the protein, retarding the rate of absorption and allowing the body to handle the aspartic acid load at a more comfortable pace. We are only concerned about the aspartic acid in our diet that can be absorbed rapidly.

The most familiar source is the low-calorie sweetener aspartame, sold under the brand names NutraSweet® and Equal®. It is easy to avoid, and my patients generally abstain from its use.

Free aspartic acid is also found in unprocessed food. Grapefruit has appreciable quantities, grapefruit juice even more. Orange juice, strawberries, nectarines, plums, and prunes (especially dried prunes) also contain considerable aspartic acid. In addition, these fruits contain significant amounts of the citrus acids, making them doubly distressing for my patients.

My patients tolerate peaches, perhaps because they contain only half the citric and malic acid of oranges, but peach juice concentrates both as well as the aspartic acid of the fruit. They are a good illustration of why my patients have to avoid any fruit juice. Tomato juice, which concentrates the tomato's low aspartic acid content plus its high glutamic acid content, is another good illustration.

Reflections

Aspartic acid came into our lives as an unwelcome guest. It made the diet more complicated for my unfortunate patients and gave them yet another dietary chemical to avoid. However, its presence provided a key to understanding both the diet and allergic disorders. It drew attention to the role of the Krebs cycle in causing allergic illness, most likely through toxic or stimulating effects on the nerves. Allergic illness due to dietary chemicals seems to result from the harmful effect of these damaged or irritated nerves.

Refined Sugar

As I recall, I was feeling pretty content. My diet was in place. It was complicated, but it worked well. At first, my patients rebelled against the elimination of favorite foods, but later they praised the diet's effectiveness. There was still much to be learned about the components of the diet—MSG, acid foods, and aspartic acid—but that was gradually happening. All in all, I was satisfied.

But there were sour notes in my symphony of contentment. Word that I was actively treating patients for food allergy with a new diet was gradually spreading among my colleagues, and they were not impressed. To allergists, patients who complain of food allergies and doctors who claim they can treat them are about as welcome as a mass murderer at a homicide detectives' convention.

After all, current thinking was that food allergy was mysterious and almost impossible to diagnose and treat. I was claiming it could be diagnosed and treated if certain dietary chemicals were avoided. Many believed that most complaints of food allergy were the wild ravings of mentally unstable patients with overstimulated imaginations. I claimed that was untrue, that my patients were right in believing they were allergic to certain foods. Current teaching insisted that food allergy was rare and could only be diagnosed by elaborate feeding and avoidance trials. I claimed it was common and could be diagnosed using patient histories and skin tests, and treated using dietary changes.

I can't say I was ostracized by my fellow allergists, but I certainly wasn't gaining their respect and admiration. The ultimate blow to my ego came when my nurses attended a lecture for nursing staff from many of the local allergy offices. The speaker poked fun of doctors who were treating food allergy by describing a local allergist who had devised a "crazy diet for his mentally unstable patients." Although the speaker didn't mention me by name, it was obvious who he was talking about. My nurses were shocked. When they told me about the incident, it became clear that my colleagues regarded my work in food allergy as falling somewhere between incompetence and quackery.

There was also another discordant note. While avoiding MSG, acidic foods, and aspartic acid was preventing headaches, diarrhea, skin rashes, and many other allergic illnesses in my patients, it wasn't preventing them all. Some patients still experienced plenty of discomfort. In the back of my mind, I knew there must be other offending foods, but the front of my mind didn't want to deal with any more additions to the diet. The back of my mind eventually won out, and another dietary chemical made its way onto the list of things to be eliminated. But only after being forcibly brought to my attention by the same friend who forced me to recognize the harmful effects of MSG.

I remember that John and I often sat at his kitchen table settling the affairs of the world and sharing personal experiences. The subject of John's dreadful cluster headaches always came up in these discussions. I wanted desperately to help him control the pain from these headaches, a searing pain he could not stop but could only relieve by inhaling pure oxygen.

We tried treating John with allergy shots and he avoided acidic foods, low-calorie sweeteners, and MSG. John was sure these dietary chemicals precipitated his dreadful cluster headaches, but since he still had a lot of them, something else *had* to be causing them. What this "something else" was eluded us—until John found it.

A New Addition to the Diet

One night as we were sitting at the table, John said, "Bill, I think I've spotted something that causes my headaches."

"Great, John. What is it?" I asked.

"Sugar."

"Oh, come on, John." I retorted in disbelief. "Lots of really elegant studies have looked at sugar and found it doesn't cause any of the illnesses popular folklore blames it for. It's even accused of making kids hyperactive and irritable, and that theory's been shot down often enough. You've got to be wrong." (Open mouth, insert foot.)

"I don't think so, Bill. I love sugar. I could eat half a pound of candy at a sitting if someone left a bowlful nearby," he confessed. "I've been wondering if the sugar might have some bearing on my headaches, so I did a little experimenting. If I have more than two sugar cookies a day, I wake up with a cluster headache, but two or less and no headache."

"John, that's hard to believe," I said, shaking my head. "This happened more then once?"

"Yes," he assured me. "Cluster headaches each time."

Now for me, an auto accident, the end of the world, and the idea of adding another chemical to the diet were equally appealing. I wasn't looking forward to telling my patients that, in addition to giving up foods high in citric acids, MSG, and aspartic acid, they'd have to avoid sweets. I could guess what their reaction would be. I also dreaded to think what my fellow allergists would say about my putting stock in the sugar-is-bad folklore. Why me?

Then I began to remember other patients who had told me they thought their headaches, diarrhea, and hives might be due to sugar. At the time, I'd dismissed their observations and even argued against them, but now I decided I should at least consider the possibility. For the next several weeks, I listened closely to my patients for signs that sugar caused their illnesses, and surprisingly the signs were there. When I asked those patients who were using the diet but were still experiencing hives, headaches, and abdominal cramps to avoid sugar, many improved remarkably. Even more amazing, their symptoms recurred when they returned to using sugar. Another chemical joined our diet!

How Can Sugar Be Harmful?

The problem with sugar is similar to that with glutamic acid and aspartic acid. Locked in protein, these amino acids do not harm my patients. Trouble erupts when my patients eat excess quantities in a rapidly absorbed or free state such as MSG or aspartame.

In most natural foods, sugar is mainly locked in storage in the form of starch. In starch, each sugar molecule is tightly bound to protein and cannot gain its freedom until digestion breaks the bonds holding it—a superb mechanism to delay the arrival of free sugar until the digestive process is ready for it. No overload. However, we ingenious humans learned to break these bonds using a process called *refining*, releasing the sweet-tasting sugar from the nearly tasteless starch. *Refined sugar* is rapidly absorbed, flooding the body with humongous numbers of sugar molecules and unleashing the illnesses that plague my patients.

Perhaps refining sugar is an example of human inventiveness outpacing our ability to tolerate the disastrous changes brought about by that inventiveness. Our metabolism was never programmed to deal with excess free sugar, and a few thousand years of evolution doesn't even come close to changing that programming.

How Does Refined Sugar Cause Illness?

Sugar is a basic supplier of energy for all animals, including humans. Its overwhelming importance in and impact on the Krebs cycle, the energy-producing process that takes place in every cell of our bodies, make it a good place to begin our search for the cause of illness, especially since the other food chemicals—MSG, citric acids, and aspartic acid—are also prominent in this cycle.

Just as gasoline is the basic fuel of the automotive engine, sugar is the fuel of the cell's energy-producing engine. Energy is released by the progressive breakdown of citric acid to succinic, fumaric, and malic acids. After the cycle is completed, sugar repairs the broken-down acid, allowing the energy cycle to start releasing energy again.

This breakdown, energy release, and repair process is extremely complex. It requires many discrete steps that are mediated by competent enzymes. If there is a weakness in any of these steps, for example, a shortage or poor functioning of an enzyme, harmful effects are likely to occur when the system is overloaded. (A case in point is that John's cluster headaches only occurred when he ate more sugar than he could tolerate.)

In discussing the other food chemicals, I pointed out evidence that these chemicals can damage nerves. The damaged nerves then activate the swelling, pain, and blockage that bring on rashes, asthma, diarrhea, and numerous other allergic illnesses. I believe the harm caused by excess sugar also may be due to its effect on nerves. This excess of sugar may have a disproportionate effect on the major nerve center of the body, the brain. Although other parts of the body accept protein and fat as well as sugar to satisfy their energy requirements, the brain accepts only sugar, which may make it especially susceptible to damage caused by sugar overload. We will discuss this point in more detail later.

Refined Sugar in the Diet

Although refined sugar does not hide in the diet, but announces its presence like a garishly painted clown, bear with me while I review some of the numerous places it can be found. Any deliciously sweet food or beverage contains sugar unless sweetened by one of the low-calorie sweeteners. A partial list includes cakes, pies, candies, sweet rolls, fudge, breakfast cereal, carbonated and noncarbonated beverages, jellies, jams, ketchup, salad dressings, ice cream, sweetened yogurt, sweetened juices, and many others. The reader will have no trouble adding to this list.

Reading the list of ingredients on processed foods and beverages will help you determine which foods are high in sugar. Food processors are required by law to list certain ingredients on the label, including sugar, with the ingredient making up the highest percentage listed first and the others listed in decreasing order. You will be surprised at the number of foods and beverages that list sugar as one of the first few ingredients.

Sugar's Many Names

Recognizing sugar can sometimes be difficult since it comes in many forms and travels under many different aliases. The following is a list of the most common ones:

Granulated sugar (refined white sugar in granulated form)
Powdered sugar (refined white sugar in powdered form)
Turbinado sugar (partially refined sugar)
Brown sugar (sugar containing molasses-flavored syrup)
Invert sugar (sugar processed with hot acid or enzymes)
Levulose or fructose (made from invert sugar)

Dextrose or corn sugar (made from invert sugar)
Lactose (milk sugar)
Maltose (sugar made from starch using yeast)
Corn syrup (partially refined starch from corn)
Molasses (partially refined sugar from plants)
Honey (refined sugar from bees)
Maple sugar and syrup (sugar from maple tree sap)

Symptoms of Sugar Intolerance

The food chemicals that bother my patients act like a gang of thieves. Each thief, by himself, might hold up a convenience store or gas station, but as a gang they might coordinate their activities to pull off the crime of the century. By working together in the gang, with each one contributing his own bit of skullduggery, they are far more powerful and destructive.

Food chemicals behave in much the same way. While my patients might have a moderate reaction to a single chemical, it is interesting to note that their symptoms are always more severe when they eat a meal high in several chemicals. The chemicals seem to *potentiate* or strengthen each others' adverse effects. Whether it is hives, wheezing, diarrhea, headaches, or another of the host of illnesses that prey on allergic people, the symptoms are far more powerful, uncomfortable, and painful.

Excess sugar affects my patients in much the same way an excess of MSG, aspartic acid, or acidic foods does. They all cause similar symptoms. In addition, like the gang of thieves where each member specializes in performing a particular crime, each of these chemicals seems to predominate in causing a particular symptom or set of symptoms.

I am extremely familiar with MSG's ability to precipitate bloating and brutal headaches (sugar also causes both, i.e., the cluster headaches John endured). I am also impressed by the ability of citric acid and its fellow acids to

provoke the itching of hives and eczema (sugar also participates). Sugar seems to have a particularly strong impact on
the nerve center of the body—the brain.

Hyperactivity and Sugar

Hyperactivity is a distressingly common and disabling
affliction. In our modern world, where education is so
highly prized, hyperactivity is a dreadful curse that
impedes the ability to learn. The hyperactive child cannot
sit still long enough to be taught, cannot remain quiet long
enough to study. Saddest of all, he or she cannot sit still
long enough for a loving parent to cuddle. Hyperactivity is
a crippling handicap.

Although most of us are aware that hyperactivity affects
many children, few realize that some adults are similarly
victimized. Like children, they are unable to remain calm
long enough to complete complex tasks or to enjoy mean-
ingful human interactions.

My patients expose me to numerous examples of food-
induced hyperactivity. A good illustration is Mary's family
of two lively little girls. By the time I walked into the examining room for our first consultation, they had partially
demolished it. Tammie was on top of the examining table,
tearing the paper to shreds, and Tracie was trying to haul
the foot stool out the door in spite of Mary's desperate
attempts to keep her from doing so.

I see hyperactivity so frequently I can spot it in an
instant. A sure sign is a child scampering around the room
like a squirrel in a cage. It's usually reinforced by a second
sign, the look on mother's face that tells me she is sorry for
the disturbance but is powerless to stop it. She *is* powerless.
You can only spank a child you love so many times before
you cannot force yourself to do it again—especially when
deep down you feel the child cannot help his or her behavior. I am one of those who believes the fault does not lie
with the child.

Mary's primary doctor sent the girls to see me because of their eczema. After testing them, we discussed the eczema, and I also raised the subject of their hyperactivity, although Mary seemed hesitant to discuss it. Like many parents of hyperactive children, she seemed to have given up hope that anything could be done about it.

We discussed dietary changes, and I stressed reduction of both acid foods (to help the eczema) and refined sugar (to see if it would have any affect on the hyperactivity). When Mary and the girls returned in three months to review their progress, she was far more willing to talk. And my office wasn't demolished.

"How did the girls like the diet, Mary?"

"Not at all, Doctor Walsh. In fact, they hate it," she admitted.

"That's not strange, Mary. Lots of our patients complain about having to avoid the foods they love. Does it help the girls?" I asked.

"It's very helpful. As long as we stick to it, their skin is almost clear."

Then she told me that the only time they had broken away from the diet was at a birthday party at school. Pop, cake, and ice cream were served, and both little girls stuffed themselves.

"Next day both were full of hives and broke out in eczema," she reported. "I was surprised at the lesson it taught them, though. Neither of them will eat acidy foods now."

I wasn't surprised. Even two- and three-year-old children will avoid sweet-tasting treats if they connect them with discomfort and pain. That's why I instruct parents not to force children to follow our diet; if the diet works and the link between food and illness is pointed out to the child, he or she will avoid the offending foods. In fact, I am often astonished by the children who intuitively avoid eating or drinking foods high in illness-producing chemicals, a habit that begins long before I first see them. If "Johnny, drink your juice" provokes a mother-child battle, there's a good possibility that Johnny and juice don't mix well.

"What about sugar, Mary?" I asked.

"That part really surprised me, Doctor Walsh. Tammie and Tracie are both much calmer on the diet. Even my mother-in-law notices, and the girls' teacher is delighted."

She told me that after the birthday party, things were pretty bad. For the next two days, the girls were unmanageable, jumping from one thing to another without stopping and driving their teacher wild. The same thing happened when Mary's father-in-law brought candy to the house.

"They got into it when we weren't watching," she said. "Now there are no more sweets at home, and their teacher watches sweets in the classroom."

The only exception I make to the "let the children manage their own diet" rule is hyperactivity. Children are often unaware of their hyperactivity, so they can't see the link between it and the diet. Patients must be aware of this cause-and-effect relationship or they won't follow the diet.

"Did you try the diet yourself, Mary?" I wondered.

"Yes, I did," she said. "As a child I was hyperactive, and now I often have days when I'm tired and irritable and can't seem to think straight. (My patients refer to this as being 'spacy' or 'spaced out'.) Now, I know I'll have days like that if I eat too much sugar. I wish someone had known about sugar and hyperactivity when I was young."

I do too. I feel sorry for the many children—and adults—who never have a chance at scholastic achievement or many of life's other rewards because of their hyperactivity. Even love and cuddling are almost impossible for children who cannot sit still long enough to be held. I firmly believe their unmanageable behavior springs not from an innate and hateful defiance, but from the hyperstimulation of the various food chemicals—especially sugar.

Mary told me she was delighted with the diet's effect on her own symptoms, but she also said it was hard for her to give up sugar. She has a genuine craving for it. In fact, when she took it out of her diet, she was miserable for five days. "I felt tired and irritable, I couldn't sleep, my hands shook, and I had a horrible headache."

Sugar Craving

Mary's experience when she eliminated sugar from her diet, what in reality were nearly intolerable withdrawal symptoms, is shared by many other patients. About one out of four or five patients crave sugar; they suffer dreadfully when they eliminate it. Their symptoms vary and may include shaky hands, muscle aches and pains, perspiration, sleeplessness, striking irritability; in other words, they feel terrible.

These withdrawal symptoms form a substantial barrier to treating patients who crave sugar. It is hard for them to recognize that sugar avoidance, which brings such pain, is necessary to control the headaches, body aches and pains, diarrhea, and other distresses that brought them to my office. When a patient craves sugar enough to suffer unpleasant withdrawal symptoms when it is eliminated, *denial* often comes into play. He or she will deny even the possibility that sugar could be causing symptoms.

It is, though. Hundreds of my patients find excess sugar causes a stuffy nose or headache; hardly a day goes by when patients fail to mention the ill effects of too many treats. My staff and I have found that any food craving is a signpost pointing to the food that is almost certainly a major cause of our patient's problems. We try to identify food cravings so we can emphasize avoiding those foods or food chemicals.

I mention food craving because we encounter it so frequently and it is so difficult to counter. In many cases, patients fight this diagnosis for years and continue to suffer until they accept it. For some odd reason, it typically takes three years for the resistant patient to come around.

A good example is Judy, a thirty-five-year-old emergency room nurse I have been treating for migraines for several years. At the outset, she tried to eliminate refined sugar, suffered overwhelming withdrawal headaches and irritability, and decided sugar was not to blame. After three years, on one of her regular follow-up visits, I asked: "How are you doing, Judy?"

"Really well, Doctor Walsh. My migraines are fine as long as I get my shots every two weeks."

"What about your diet? I asked. "Do any foods bring on the headaches?"

"I have to avoid tomatoes, oranges, and MSG entirely or I get bad headaches," she said. "I also have to watch potatoes and cheese, and I can only have pizza if I don't eat any bad food for two days before the pizza."

When I asked, "What about sugar?" I was surprised at Judy's answer.

"I've eliminated it from my diet altogether. Once I start to eat sugar, I can't stop and I end up irritable, I can't think clearly, and get hit with a horrible headache."

You do not make friends when you say "I told you so," so I didn't. But I remembered three years back when Judy said the diet was stupid and sugar didn't bother her. Eventually she became convinced sugar was the culprit, but she suffered a long time before recognizing it. Perhaps her story will help others with sugar craving realize their problem.

A Reflection

I often reflect on my experiences with sugar. I was reluctant to add it to the elimination diet because it would be yet another chemical that my patients must avoid. However, together my patients and I learned it must be eliminated to truly control their distressing symptoms. Sugar's effects on the brain—sugar craving, hyperactivity, 'spacy thinking'— also forced me to confront the effect of all allergies, especially the food chemical allergies, on the central nervous system. It is this connection that ensures its permanent place in the diet.

Other Foods and Beverages

In our discussion of foods and beverages that cause my patients' reactions, I touched only lightly on several that merit further consideration. In addition, there are a few others that ought to be discussed. These foods and beverages are major components of our diet, and sensitive patients must be extremely cautious when consuming them. We will examine them more thoroughly in this chapter, as well as addressing some issues frequently raised by patients for whom I prescribe the elimination diet.

Corn

Corn deserves special attention because it is so prevalent in our modern diet and also because it is often a major problem. For many of our patients, corn provokes the same symptoms as the dietary chemicals—sugar, acidic foods, MSG, and aspartic acid. This is somewhat of an enigma because when these patients are skin tested to corn, the test is negative. This indicates that the protein in corn is not to blame (allergy to protein is the usual cause of a positive skin test), but that the reaction is more likely amino acid related.

Today's corn plant was hybridized from an American weed used for food thousands of years ago. This evolution changed it from an ear the size of a strawberry to the seed-bearing hulk grown on modern farms today. As each generation of seed was selected for its increased size, it must also have been cultivated for taste. We know that MSG gives both natural and processed foods a robust and pleasant taste, and corn is naturally rich in this free amino acid. Regrettably, the high MSG content that accounts for the pleasant taste sought by our ancestors is probably also responsible for the unpleasant reactions my patients suffer.

The ramifications of corn allergy are disturbing. Corn, which is the world's most widely distributed food crop, is found in countless products, including breakfast cereals, corn meal, many varieties of canned corn, corn bread, corn on the cob, corn starch, corn syrup, crackers, popcorn, tortillas and numerous others. Obviously, eliminating corn from the diet poses a terrible hardship. A frequent question my patients ask is whether they most avoid all corn products.

While I can't be entirely sure, I don't think so. MSG decomposes at 250 degrees Fahrenheit, and any product processed at a higher temperature presumably will be low in intact MSG. Therefore, unless MSG is added after baking, cereals, crackers, breads, and similar products are probably acceptable for patients who are allergic to chemicals.

Unfortunately, the temperature of boiling water is only 212 degrees Fahrenheit, so foods prepared in this way generally cannot be expected to be free of MSG. This must be the reason so many of my patients find that corn on the cob causes them grief. The anticipation with which we await the late summer harvest of delicious sweet corn, and the widespread popularity of this grain product, combine to obscure its obnoxious effects on my patients. They are often unaware that they are allergic to corn until we warn them to watch for symptoms after they eat it.

I share my patients' love of corn on the cob and their distress after eating it. In fact, the bloating and abdominal pains I was beset with after a delicious meal of corn on the cob first brought this food allergy to my attention.

Unfortunately, the potential for corn on the cob to cause suffering is shared by popcorn. I suspect that even the relatively high temperature required to pop corn is not sufficient to destroy the high levels of MSG.

If corn is cut from the cob and then boiled, my patients often seem able to tolerate it. With this preparation method, each of the corn seeds is cut open, which apparently allows the MSG to be dissolved and dissipated into the boiling water. Another way to reduce MSG in foods is to store them for at least twenty-four hours before preparation; stored foods contain less MSG then fresh foods.

Peanuts

I feel terrible when I tell my patients they should avoid popcorn because it often brings on reactions such as headaches, diarrhea, rashes, and the myriad other illnesses that plague the susceptible allergic patient. I feel even worse telling them that peanuts can cause the same distressing symptoms.

I know that many patients would more readily accept the need to avoid popcorn if they could substitute a crunchy handful of peanuts as they watch a ball game or snack at a party. Unfortunately for many patients, this substitution brings regrettable symptoms.

My staff and I learned about the potential for peanuts to cause harm from patients who gave up popcorn when they found it caused them to feel sick. Many of them told us that when they replaced popcorn with peanuts, they experienced the same discomfort.

It is surprising that pain and discomfort can be caused by such an important food source. Like corn, peanuts are a major food crop; seventeen million metric tons are grown per year and processed as peanut butter or simply roasted and sold at sporting events, circuses, etc., and as at-home snacks. Also like corn, the peanut has long been used as a human food. It is known to have existed as early as 950 B.C. in South America, and its use was widespread throughout Mexico and South America when early explorers reached these areas in the sixteenth century.

The peanut may be similar to corn in another way. Although I was unable to determine the exact MSG content of the peanut from my reference materials, I suspect that as a member of the pea family (hence the name *pea*nut), it is likely to be high in MSG. In fact, peas contain more MSG than corn. Since most of my patients tolerate boiled peas, this process must reduce the level of MSG, but unfortunately, the processing of shelled and unshelled peanuts does not seem to have similar benefits.

Oddly enough, many of my patients who cannot eat a handful of peanuts do seem to tolerate peanut butter. Perhaps the process for making peanut butter takes place at temperatures high enough to destroy MSG. We tell our patients to try eating peanut butter if they miss it in their diet; they can continue to use it as long as it does not stimulate symptoms.

A word of caution: *People who experience life-threatening symptoms (i.e., breathing difficulty, hives, loss of consciousness, or other severe reactions) from eating peanuts should never try to eat this food in any form.*

Alcoholic Beverages

Another issue our patients want to know about is consumption of alcoholic beverages. Unfortunately, because distillers and wine producers are not required to provide any information on liquor labels other than alcohol content, my advice about alcoholic beverages is based on meager data. However, certain facts can serve as a partial guide to their use.

As mentioned earlier, because fermentation of any food or beverage releases MSG as the protein breaks down, you can expect to find MSG in any alcoholic beverage. My primary advice is to drink in moderation so that you do not accumulate an excess of MSG.

Some alcoholic beverages seem worse than others. Corn-based liquors such as bourbon cause my patients great distress; they seem to tolerate grain-based beverages such as scotch much better. The same is true for beer. American beer is often brewed from corn and seems to be poorly tolerated by my patients compared to barley-based beers such as the German ales and lagers.

I also caution my patients to avoid using any mix other then water; these products usually contain high amounts of sugar and acid.

Another piece of advice I give my patients is to be extremely careful of wines and brandy. Because both are fermented from grapes and are high in both citric and tartaric acid as well as MSG, they are particularly bothersome to my patients, especially the red wines. I recommend asking for a glass of water instead.

Yogurt

Yogurt is produced from milk by fermenting it with two bacteria. Unfortunately, this fermentation probably releases the glutamic and aspartic acids that are bound to the milk's protein, and both of these acids are irritating to my patients. The amount of these free amino acids probably varies depending on the fermentation process, as is the case with cheese; the more fermented (aged) the cheese, the more elevated the MSG content. Lacking information on the free amino acid content of various yogurt brands, it is impossible to tell which may be lowest in these acids and thus best for my patients.

Since I do not believe yogurt contains particularly high levels of aspartic acid and MSG, I believe most of my patients can tolerate a limited amount in their diet; however, eating a lot of it would be a great mistake. It would also be inadvisable to eat flavored yogurts, especially those that contain aspartame; the sugar and acid content combined with MSG and aspartic acid could be overwhelming.

The Cabbage Family

I am surprised by the number of my patients who are sensitive to cabbage, cauliflower, broccoli, and brussels sprouts. My nursing staff and I took an informal survey and found that the majority of our patients suffer symptoms from either corn or the cabbage family. Interestingly enough, most patients reacted to one or the other, but not to both. I have no idea why this is so, nor do I know why so many react to the cabbage family. Watch for this allergy. Boiling these foods well may allow you to eat them if you react to them when they are uncooked.

Vitamins

The question my patients ask most frequently is: "If I cut out all these foods, where do I get my vitamins?" The fact is that when you examine the foods that are acceptable on the diet, the answer is obvious. The many fresh fruits, vegetables, and meats that are allowed contain all the vitamins you need for proper nutrition. And conversely, many of the foods we recommend eliminating are not high in nutritional value.

Many people supplement their diet with extra vitamins, in most cases, the one-a-day type. For most of my patients, this is unwise; supplemental vitamins often make them ill. I confess to doing this from time to time, but a week of taking vitamins makes me so sick I am cured of the temptation.

I am not sure why vitamin supplements cause so much discomfort. One possible explanation is that they usually contain citric acid. Pharmacists tell me that vitamin C needs to be combined with citric acid to prevent deterioration and inactivation, but this is only a partial answer. Many of my patients also react poorly to vitamins that do not contain vitamin C.

The fact that so many of my patients suffer bloating, diarrhea, rashes, abdominal pain, and a number of other symptoms from taking vitamins makes me wonder whether we should reexamine the value of these dietary supplements. They may not be as harmless as we think. It's like the owner of a Volkswagen "Beetle" who isn't satisfied with its ruggedness and reliability, but also wants it to accelerate like a dragster, so he drives it to the airport and fills the tank with jet engine fuel. Much to his chagrin, he finds that instead of accelerating better, the car barely operates at all because it was never designed to run on jet fuel.

Maybe vitamins are like jet fuel for our bodies. Instead of improving its operation, do they pose a threat we aren't even aware of?

Illnesses Caused by Food Allergy

Describing the illnesses caused by food allergy is like trying to gift-wrap an elephant—there's not enough paper to do it. What's more, even if you had enough paper, where would you start?

Now I know this analogy is a little ridiculous, but it does give you some idea of the dilemma I faced in writing this chapter. Food allergy provokes so many illnesses that to include an elaborate scientific description of all of them would have made this book so expensive the average person couldn't afford it. Besides that, I did not write this book to help you diagnose your own illnesses. Diagnosing and treating illnesses should be left to your doctor, and you should not rely on any book to diagnose yourself. Your doctor is trained to recognize symptoms and determine their cause. Go to him for help so you can avoid the mistakes that will surely result from self-diagnosis and treatment.

Instead, the purpose of this book is simply to make you more conscious of food allergy and the many illnesses associated with it. The summary of allergic illnesses in this chapter is intended to increase your awareness of their symptoms. If you are experiencing any of these symptoms, you should at least consider the possibility that they are food-related.

One way to comprehend the multitude of these ailments is to consider how food allergy causes harm. I believe allergenic foods, especially food chemicals, disrupt the Krebs cycle, the basic energy-producing sequence that supplies all the cells of the body—all the muscles, bones, skin, blood vessels, and other organs that are so essential to life. Any disruption of this process will have widespread consequences.

The Krebs cycle also energizes our nerves. Earlier I presented evidence that the discomfort and pain of allergic illness results from damage to the nerves, damage caused by an overload of the chemicals involved in the production of nerve energy. Nerves stimulate and control virtually every area of the body, so by damaging nerves, food allergy can wreak havoc anywhere in the body. It uses nerves as pathways to various parts of the body, just as we use highways to travel from one place to another. That's why my patients suffer multiple symptoms simultaneously, symptoms that make food allergy difficult to pin down because they seem to be unconnected. However, they are related through the body's intricate network of nerves.

The long list of disorders for which food allergy is the *direct cause* is augmented by numerous illnesses for which it is *indirectly responsible*. Like an inconsiderate bully, allergy seems delighted by the opportunity to further torment my patients who have non-allergy-related disease. For instance, we often see patients with back pain due to degenerated vertebrae or whiplash injury that is greatly intensified by food allergy. For patients with intestinal inflammations such as ulcerative colitis, allergy makes their bouts of painful diarrhea much more severe. In these instances, the disorder is not directly caused by food allergy, but the *preexisting condition is aggravated* by it.

In the following summary of allergic illnesses, I won't make a point of telling you which are direct and which are indirect. Since doctors are unsure of the cause of many illnesses, it isn't important to make that distinction. The important thing is that if exposure to certain food chemicals is causing discomfort and pain, those chemicals must be avoided.

Allergic Illnesses—The Blood Vessels

The blood vessels are an appropriate place to begin our exploration of the illnesses brought on by food allergy. So many allergic symptoms can be explained in part or altogether by swelling or spasm of the blood vessels.

MIGRAINE HEADACHE. A popular theory for what causes **migraine** is that it is related to spasms of the blood vessels in the head. The resulting restriction of blood flow denies blood-borne nutrition and oxygen to the brain and eyes. This decrease in energy and oxygen produces the vision changes and numbness that warn many patients they are about to be socked with migraine's agonizing pain.

The pain occurs when the blood vessels relax because they are tired of being in spasm. Unfortunately, they relax too much and swell like a boiling sausage; the pulsating blood flowing through them stretches pain fibers, and a throbbing headache ensues.

HIVES AND ANGIOEDEMA. Anther disorder that can be explained by blood vessel changes is **hives**, a condition characterized by intensely itchy red blotches—some large, some small—caused by the swelling of small blood vessels at the surface of the skin. The swollen vessels leak fluid into the surrounding skin, causing the hives to break out. The discomfort that accompanies the hives results from irritation of the itch-sensitive nerves at the skin's surface. Not only are hives uncomfortable, they can be terribly embarrassing. Imagine going to work with red splotches all over your face!

Angioedema is a condition in which the hives form deep in the skin. Patients develop swelling that can turn fingers into sausages, raise flat-topped welts on the skin, or puff up the eyelids, hands, and feet. These deep-seated swellings, which are sometimes redder and sometimes paler than the surrounding skin, typically do not itch because the nerve fibers at the surface of the skin are not stimulated to send out an itch sensation. Often hives and angioedema strike together, and my patients suffer both the red, itchy hives and the uncomfortable swelling.

ASTHMA. Blood vessel changes can also explain some characteristics of **asthma**, which causes difficulty in clearing air from the lungs. During severe asthma attacks, the chests of victims become distended because their breath is trapped in their lungs like the air in an overinflated balloon. Exhaling, which is second nature to those without asthma, becomes an exhausting struggle.

Breathing is difficult because the passages that carry air to the far reaches of the lungs are obstructed. The blood vessels swell and leak fluid into the airway lining, much as they do in hives and angioedema. The swollen linings partially block the passage of air, producing the frightening whistle or wheezing sound that is so familiar in asthma sufferers.

The same swelling that causes hives, asthma, and migraine headaches can occur in a number of other areas. Next we'll examine the consequences of this reaction in the respiratory tract, the sinuses, the chest cavity, and the joints.

SWELLING IN THE RESPIRATORY TRACT. If the swelling centers in the vocal cords, it can cause **hoarseness and loss of voice**. This is a frequent complaint of many of my patients, especially singers, ministers, and others who frequently address the public. Perhaps the strain these activities put on their vocal cords weakens the area and makes it more susceptible to the voice changes caused by allergy.

Swelling in this same area, especially when accompanied by an annoying itch, can lead to the **chronic cough** and **persistent throat clearing** that exasperates so many of my patients. The spring and fall rainy seasons send a constant stream of coughing and throat-clearing patients to my office, usually at the request of parents, spouses, or friends who are tired of listening to this irritating noise day and night.

For a sizable share of the population, the airway swelling is so pronounced that they can actually strangle! They experience an **obstruction of the airway**—a swelling that makes it extremely difficult for them to breathe. Fortunately the strangling has not been fatal in any of my patients because the swelling has caused only a partial blockage. Needless to say, they live in fear that one of these attacks will be their last.

This frightening disorder is often misdiagnosed as hyperventilation by doctors who are unaware of this surprisingly frequent allergic reaction. Patients who suffer from angioedema in the airway usually know that something is blocking their breathing, and will even point to the spot on the neck or chest where they feel the obstruction. Their struggle for air is similar to the **hyperventilation** that accompanies anxiety attacks, but in these cases, the anxiety is brought on by the condition instead being the cause of it. Forget the tranquilizers!

When angioedema occurs higher in the respiratory tract, its symptoms are relatively harmless but unpleasant. If the swelling is at the back of the throat, it can cause recurrent **sore throats**. Although painful to my patients, these sore throats seem to have no infectious basis because they produce negative throat cultures. It can also produce **swelling of the tongue, lips, or membranes in the mouth**, as well as the most common complaint of allergy patients—**nasal stuffiness**. This unpleasant symptom, which results from swelling in the mucous membranes of the nose, is like having a constant cold with its accompanying tiredness, irritability, and just plain yuckiness. It is very frustrating to treat this condition if the patient refuses to limit the foods and beverages that promote the stuffiness.

SINUS HEADACHE. If the swelling is even higher in the respiratory tract—in the sinuses—my patients experience the nagging, steady pressure and pain of **sinus headache**. Over half of the patients who come to us for treatment have aggravating pain in the forehead, eyes, cheeks, or back of the head that is characteristic of these distressing headaches. I know firsthand how distressful they can be since I used to suffer dreadful sinus headaches. The opportunity to help others avoid these headaches is one of the things that attracted me to the field of allergy.

SWELLING IN THE CHEST. Another surprisingly common allergic symptom is **chest pain**. My patients often complain of a painful tightening or heavy sensation under the sternum (breastbone), much like that experienced by people who are having heart attacks. I imagine more than a few doctors have been surprised to have an allergic patient with severe chest pain produce a normal EKG.

SWELLING IN THE JOINTS. Since allergy is known to be a tormentor of weak or damaged areas, it is no surprise that angioedema frequently attacks the muscles and joints of patients with non-allergy-related diseases such as **rheumatoid arthritis** or **osteoarthritis**. The swelling generally occurs deep in the affected joints and is barely noticeable on the surface of the skin, producing little or no heat or redness (heat and redness are the hallmarks of arthritic inflammation). Many of my patients with arthritis experience episodes of pain in their arthritic joints when they do not watch their diet.

This same annoying pain bothers joints that have been damaged by injury. Patients with **whiplash** and other spine injury are vulnerable, as well as those with **TMJ** or **post-**

traumatic joint injury (for example, joints damaged by football injury). Here again I speak from personal experience. My "football" knee aches and swells with fluid when I exceed my tolerance for food chemicals—in my case, almost always MSG blundered into by mistake.

NERVES, BLOOD VESSELS, AND MYSTERY. Much of the mystery surrounding allergies seems to stem from the fact that they strike such widely separated areas of the body, areas as unrelated as the joints and respiratory tract. But in the previous discussion, we used a *key bit of information* to dispel this mystery.

We saw how widely separated and unrelated parts of the body are affected by the same process—swelling and spasm of blood vessels. In tracking this swelling as it moved around the body, we learned why different allergic disorders bring discomfort and pain. We also saw that areas already weakened by injury or disease as well as genetically predisposed areas can be vulnerable to allergy attack.

Now that we know allergy is not really mysterious, let's explore the relationship between the blood vessels and nerves that have been damaged by the overload of dietary chemicals.

THE RELATIONSHIP. Blood vessels can no more dilate or spasm by themselves than a car can drive itself. Imagine picking up the morning paper and reading:

MR. JONES'S 1990 HUPMOBILE JAILED AFTER BEING CONVICTED OF SMASHING INTO STOP SIGN

Upon reading this, whoever is in charge would probably make reservations for the reporter, the judge, and the arresting officer on the nearest psychiatric ward and order a trial for Mr. Jones, the car's driver.

Just as cars do not drive themselves, blood vessels do not order themselves to dilate. Nerves do, and understanding this relationship is key to understanding the effects of allergic reactions on the nerves and blood vessels.

In an earlier discussion, I presented evidence that nerves are damaged by allergy and that these damaged nerves may stimulate blood vessels to swell and leak. However, I did not mention that in addition to nerve damage, there is another mechanism that may stimulate the vessel-swelling commands of nerves.

Many of the nerves in the blood vessels are stimulated by *neurotransmitters* (chemicals that transmit or carry messages to nerves). Both MSG and the aspartic acid in low-calorie sweeteners are known neurotransmitters; in fact, they are also neurostimulating and neurotoxic (damaging to nerves). I think it is logical to assume that sugar and acidic foods are likewise damaging to nerves because they cause the same illnesses in my patients. It is possible—even probable—that the rapid absorption of these chemicals leads to blood levels that directly stimulate the nerves that govern blood vessels, forcing dilatation and swelling and provoking my patient's discomfort and pain.

Effect of Allergic Illness on Smooth Muscle

Blood vessels are not the only body tissue involved in allergic illnesses. Smooth muscle also participates.

THE SAME MECHANISM. Allergy's effect on smooth muscle is the same as on blood vessels. Like the vessels, smooth muscle is richly supplied with nerves, and these nerves "drive" smooth muscle like we drive a car. Also like blood vessels, nerve impulses force smooth muscle to spasm or relax. Unlike the vessels, which cause allergic illness by relaxation (swelling), allergic suffering occurs when smooth muscle spasms or contracts. The smooth muscles we are concerned with encircle the digestive tract and the airways of the lung.

ASTHMA. In looking at asthma, we saw that blood vessel swelling in the lining of the airways constricts the air passages, obstructing the flow of air and causing the whistling or wheezing sound we hear as the air forces itself out of these narrowed air passages. But we shouldn't limit our discussion to swelling of the lining because it is not the only reason the air passages constrict.

Each passage is surrounded by layers of muscle, called smooth muscle, like the water running to a sprinkler is surrounded by the walls of a hose. Unlike the rigid walls of a hose, the muscle around the air passages is alive and in constant motion, contracting and dilating to open or close the numerous branches of the airway, directing the flow of air to different parts of the lung like a traffic officer directs the flow of traffic through a busy intersection.

What if during the rush hour, the traffic officer went on strike, closing half of each road leading into the intersection? Pandemonium would result, with angry, snarling drivers trapped in a gridlock. The stream of traffic would be slowed almost to a halt, and it would take forever for the cars to thread their way through the intersection.

Asthma is like that. Things go smoothly when the airway muscle is functioning normally, contracting and relaxing as it calmly directs the flow of air. When the muscle is in spasm during an asthma attack, the airway narrows, restricting the flow of air through every intersection of the lung.

Food allergy is only one of many causes of asthma attacks, but when the diet is involved, the most likely reason is nerve malfunction signaling the smooth muscle of the airways to go into spasm. Dietary discretion can control this spasm the same way it controls the blood vessel swelling in the lining of the airway.

SMOOTH MUSCLE SPASM ALONG THE DIGESTIVE TRACT. Spasm in the esophagus, one of the first muscles to come in contact with dietary chemicals, causes a distressing **chest pain** similar to the pain that accompanies angioedema as well as to that associated with heart attack. Spasm can also cause transient **difficulties in swallowing**. My patients frequently experience these symptoms.

When such pain occurs in the stomach, it is referred to as **acid stomach** and often leads patients to suspect that they have an ulcer. Those who do have ulcers are especially susceptible to this condition, another example of allergy preying upon an already weakened area. The combination of food allergy and ulcer produces a persistent, knawing pain. Unfortunately, changing the diet will not cure an ulcer, but it can eliminate this aggravating complication.

At the end of the intestine, and surrounded by the same smooth muscle, is the colon, an organ frequently affected by allergy. Here muscle spasms give rise to the **abdominal cramps and diarrhea** that so often make my patients' lives miserable. **Spastic colon** is a frequent diagnosis given to my patients. In most cases, food allergy is not suspected; however, the effects of spastic colon are usually alleviated by changing the diet.

I first encountered this problem years ago in a sensitive and proud woman whose life was terribly affected by diarrhea. Whenever she and her husband went out with friends to dinner and a show, they went an hour early. The reason? She would have an hour-long bout with diarrhea immediately following the meal. Before they could proceed to the theater, her husband and their companions had to wait patiently while she suffered through what must have been a very mortifying situation.

I still remember her sad story, and I regret that I didn't understand food allergy then as well as I do now. At the time, I didn't know how to control her diarrhea.

Allergic Illness—Contact Dermatitis

Our trip through the digestive tract ends at the rectum, where an uncommon but miserable effect of food chemicals manifests itself. A small number of allergy-prone adults complain of an intense **rectal itching** that mystifies doctors. The acidic foods seem unusually adept at causing this uncomfortable and embarrassing condition, although the other chemicals also contribute. **Diaper rash** in babies is more common and is often caused by these same offenders. I suspect that as the stool passes through the anus, the high concentration of diet chemicals it contains irritate and burn the skin. We know this contact reaction occurs at the other end of the body, where our patients suffer a **scalp rash** marked by itching and sores from using shampoos that contain citrus. (I am not sure of the propriety of discussing scalp and rectal rashes in the same paragraph, but they are related.)

Another form of contact dermatitis that should be mentioned is the oh-so-common **hand dermatitis**, sometimes called housewife's hand dermatitis. Anyone who handles acidic foods is susceptible. Contact with these foods reinforces the dermatitis-producing effect of consuming food chemicals (making hands red, dry, cracked, and pathetically itchy).

Allergic Illness—The Central Nervous System

The effect of food allergy on the central nervous system (the brain) is perhaps the most difficult subject to discuss because it is surrounded by uncertainty and controversy. Many doctors and laypeople do not accept the idea that food chemicals can impair brain function or be responsible for the many symptoms our patients suffer. They believe anxiety, depression, and other mood disorders are more likely to be at the root of these symptoms.

I disagree. As we examined our modern diet, we found that certain components are known neurotoxins (aspartic and glutamic acids) and saw how they and their fellow rogue chemicals can generate allergic disease through injury to nerves. Do we suddenly reverse our thinking when it comes to the major nerve center of the body, the brain? I see no reason to do so.

At the same time, I don't want you to think that food chemicals are solely or even primarily responsible for these disorders. Anxiety and psychological instability may be major causes, or they may be contributing factors that potentiate allergy's harm. However, in many cases, food allergy seems to drive these illnesses like a hammer drives a nail, while in other cases, it seems to play more of a supportive role, like the fingers holding the nail. But whatever the relative contribution of each factor, the important thing is to gain relief for my patients, and I find that changing the diet often provides that relief.

A Patient's Story

Perhaps the best way to illustrate the effects of food allergy on mental function is through one of my patient histories. Frequently I see patients who complain of allergic symptoms that are so minor I wonder why they came, but when I ask them how they feel in general, the real reason comes tumbling out. They tell me about being tired, irritable, and depressed all the time—just plain feeling crummy and unable to cope with everyday life. Jackie is one of those patients.

A woman in her forties, Jackie is a middle manager in a nationally known company. She had been feeling tired and listless for so long she was worried about her ineffectiveness at work. "I had my doctor check my thyroid because I was sure I was hypothyroid, but the tests were normal. Then I began to think that I was 'wimping out'—that the tiredness was all in my head."

"That's not at all unusual, Jackie," I assured her. "It isn't necessarily all in your head. Many people find physical factors, such as food allergy, cause these symptoms."

Jackie's symptoms are as frequent in my patients as stuffy nose or headache. What's more, patient's often hide these symptoms as they would hide a disgraceful family secret. Like Jackie, they are afraid to "wimp out" because they don't want to be thought of as a hypochondriac—a whiner and a complainer. They are not any of these things. **Tiredness, irritability,** and often **hyperactivity** (the inability to concentrate) are very real, very common companions of food allergy and usually respond to diet changes.

When Jackie returned to my office after her first three months of treatment to tell me what happened when she changed her diet, we had the following conversation.

"How are you doing, Jackie?"

"Changing my diet helped much more then I thought it would, Doctor Walsh," she reported. "I know you asked me to retry the foods I've eliminated, but I feel so good, I'm afraid to return to them."

"How has the diet made a difference?" I asked.

"I'm surprised at how much better I feel. I'm not as tired, and I've got a lot more ambition at work. Although I'm not a hundred percent better, I have improved so much I no longer think it's all in my head."

Then Jackie told me about another interesting discovery she had made. "I was talking to one of my coworkers the other day. She told me she sees you, too, and has to follow the same diet. Every time she cheats, she ends up feeling tired and irritable and unproductive at work."

Since then, Jackie has found that her ability to concentrate at work is also affected when she strays from the diet, a symptom shared by many of my patients. They have a hard time describing this familiar result of exposure to dietary chemicals, but many agree that an appropriate label would be **"spacy" thinking.**

I know you might think this is going too far—that foods we have eaten all our lives can't possibly affect our mental ability—but don't be too sure. We are learning that the thought and memory processes that take place in the brain are assisted and influenced by neurotransmitters. It does not require a great stretch of imagination to reason that the *neurostimulatory* and *neurotoxic neurotransmitter* chemicals in our modern diet may muddle our thinking and turn it "spacy."

Neurotransmitters are a hot research topic in the study of **depression**. Since allergy and depression are both frequent in the population, it isn't surprising that they often coexist in our patients. Food allergy does not cause depression, but the tiredness, irritability, and ineffective thinking that often accompany it can make depression much harder to overcome. Modifying the diet can help tremendously. Depressed patients who also happen to be allergy-prone deserve the same care as those who are free of this debilitating illness.

Other Allergic Illnesses

Although I have described many of my patient's discomforts and pains, there are still many others I have not included. Every day patients tell me of aches, pains, and discomforts brought on by allergy, many strange and unusual, all a burden. The reason I have not mentioned them is not that they are unimportant, but that there are so many.

Putting Food Allergy in Perspective

What if the president of the United States were to suddenly address the nation in these words:

> "My fellow Americans, our country faces a crisis of unimaginable severity. Not enough scientists and engineers are being trained to design the new machines our modern age demands, or to run the factories that manufacture those machines. Because we lack people who are trained in these skills, we are falling behind competitively in the world marketplace. This must change.

> "Therefore, Congress has passed into law, and I have signed, an emergency measure to reverse this unacceptable situation. From now on, all children will study to be engineers and scientists. The only courses offered in grade school, high school, and college will be math and science. No more English, history, social studies, or business classes will be allowed."

Can you imagine the outrage this misguided proclamation would be greeted with? No doubt a whole new protest movement would form overnight, and with good reason. We all know that not everyone has the talent or the inclination to be an engineer or a scientist, and that our society could not prosper without writers, historians, social scientists, or business experts. It would be a mistake to force everyone into the same profession.

Surprisingly, this scenario has great pertinence to my patients and their food allergies. Just as it is a mistake to think that all children are alike, it is wrong to think that all patients are alike, or to think that all allergic illnesses are identical.

Each patient is a special individual with a distinctive illness that is not like any other patient's illness. For instance, food allergy is an overwhelmingly important cause of headache or wheezing for some patients; for others, food allergy is only a minor contributing factor. Some patients may react badly to one food, while others may be able to tolerate that same food but will have a severe reaction to another food. To keep food allergy in perspective, a doctor must remember these differences in patients, illnesses, and causes. To do otherwise would be a great mistake.

How does a doctor or layman approach the diagnosis and treatment of food allergy and keep it in perspective? I do it by following a number of principles I have learned over many years from the magnificent patients who worked with me to control their discomfort and pain. Each patient's problems and response to treatment helped to slowly open the door to the secrets of allergy. (Perhaps the door will never be fully open, nor the secrets fully revealed.) Let's look at the principles I use to put food allergy in perspective.

NO ILLNESS IS ALLERGY UNTIL IT IS DIAGNOSED AS SUCH BY YOUR PRIMARY PHYSICIAN. Not all illness is due to allergy. You do not need an allergist to do skin tests for your headaches if they are due to a brain lesion, or skin testing for diarrhea if you have bowel disease. Go to your primary doctor for diagnosis. Go to an allergist only after obtaining a proper primary diagnosis.

A NONALLERGIC ILLNESS DOES NOT PRECLUDE ALLERGY. This principle is not a contradiction of the first one. I treat many patients with brain lesions for the allergic component of their headaches, and I help patients with bowel inflammation alleviate the part of their cramps and diarrhea that is caused by allergy. They deserve the same care as any other allergic patient.

NEVER IGNORE ENVIRONMENTAL ALLERGY IN DIAGNOSING FOOD ALLERGY. It is best to assume (and probably true) that all patients react to both foods and to the dust, mold, pollen, and pets in their environment. Patients both breathe and eat; to focus on one to the exclusion of the other means the patient's illness will not be fully evaluated. It is tempting to focus only on food allergy when investigating the allergic reactions of some patients. For example, we often see patients who react to a specific food (i.e., shrimp) in a specific way (i.e., hives). The obvious diagnosis is food allergy, solo and uncomplicated.

Not necessarily. To understand this point, visualize a patient as a bucket you want to fill. If the bucket is already full, any added water will slop over the side. If it's empty, you can add a lot of water before it spills over. The water represents food allergy, and the water spilling over the side is the allergic reaction. Sometimes a patient's food allergy is super strong, and just like adding water to a bucket that is filled to the brim will always cause it to overflow, eating the offending food will always lead to a reaction. All by itself.

At other times, the food allergy is only moderately—or even mildly—strong (like a cup of water poured into the bucket). The patient must be primed or prepared to react before the food can cause trouble, just as the bucket must be almost full before water spills over the side.

This principle explains why food allergy is so frequently intermittent. On a particular day, sugar provokes a migraine; on another day, no headache. Perhaps on the day of the headache, the patient was exposed to a large amount of dust while cleaning out the basement, plus the ragweed pollen count was high. In this example, environmental allergy primed my patient for a headache brought on by sugar, a headache that would not occur on a day with low dust and ragweed exposure.

Dust, mold, and pollen often prime patients to react to foods. That's why categorizing any food allergy as "solo and uncomplicated" is frequently a mistake if environmental allergy is ignored. Foods are usually not the only cause of allergy, even in cases where the evidence points overwhelmingly in that direction.

NEVER IGNORE FOOD ALLERGY IN DIAGNOSING ENVIRONMENTAL ALLERGY. This principle is the inverse of the previous one. Just as it is a mistake to ignore the influence of the environment on food allergy, it is also a mistake to ignore the influence of foods on environmental allergy. Patients suffer if their doctor errs in either direction.

But what about the patient with solo, uncomplicated pollen allergy, the patient who sneezes only during the grass pollen season? Surely foods aren't the cause of this sneezing.

For an answer, let's pretend the allergic patient must carry his allergies around in a bucket. For many, grass (or tree or ragweed) pollen allergy fills the bucket to overflowing. But is the overflow a trickle, or is it a flood? If the patient's bucket is empty of any other allergy, chances are it's a trickle. But if the bucket is partially filled with food allergies, even though the bucket doesn't overflow during the pollen-free months, when the pollen allergy is added, there is likely to be a flood. Similarly, my patients with pollen allergy can be far more uncomfortable if they eat certain foods when the pollen count is high.

Allergy to the food chemicals is so common in our patients that my nurses and I routinely look for them when we investigate problems due to pollen, dust, mold, and pet allergy. The single act of changing the diet during the time my patient is suffering from something in the environment often determines the success or failure of our treatment. It can change a flood of allergy misery into a trickle of discomfort, a miserable pollen season into one that is merely uncomfortable.

EXPLORE BOTH FOOD AND ENVIRONMENTAL ALLERGY IN EVERY PATIENT. This principle reinforces the previous two. A patient is ill served by the doctor who ignores food allergy and concentrates on environmental causes such as pollen, dust, mold, and pets, or vice versa. Breathing and eating are so basic to our existence that factors which affect either area can be equally detrimental to our quality of life. Therefore, it is essential to question the influence of the pollen season on food allergy and of food sensitivity on pollen allergies. Patients deserve these answers.

ATTACK OVERPOWERING FOOD ALLERGY BY ATTACKING ENVIRONMENTAL ALLERGY. Often a patient's food allergies are uncomplicated and easy to diagnose, and avoidance of one or several foods solves the problem neatly. However, sometimes patients are allergic to so many foods and suffer such devastating reactions, I feel almost powerless to help them.

Many examples spring to mind—patients with food allergy so universal they are allergic to practically every food and beverage in our modern diet. Some of the most tragic and pitiable of these patients are those with bulimia and anorexia nervosa. Their horrendous food allergies make these formidable illnesses even more resistant to treatment.

The only effective way to treat these seemingly hopeless cases of food allergy is to eliminate as many other allergens as possible. Using the analogy of the bucket, if the patient's food allergy causes it to overflow, the logical solution is to ensure the bucket is empty of any other allergic factors to make more room for food allergy. In other words, reduce the flood to a trickle.

In this approach to allergy care, the most important strategy is not the treatment of the food allergy itself but the aggressive treatment of any environmental allergy the patient may have—no matter how small. It is amazing how well this works.

ACID FOODS, MSG, ASPARTIC ACID, AND SUGAR ARE THE MOST IMPORTANT FOOD ALLERGIES. This principle downplays the importance of common food allergies such as milk, wheat, peanut butter, and all the other foods that cause allergic symptoms. Since these food allergies are usually spotted by the patient, parents, or primary doctor, the diagnosis is usually apparent, the treatment is avoidance, and an allergist is seldom needed.

Not so with the patients I see. They are part of an immense group of sufferers who react to multiple foods. Diagnosing them is baffling, treating them is complicated, and the skills of an allergist are usually required. For these patients, the potent and damaging food chemicals are commonly the direct or indirect causes of illness, and treatment will fail unless their use of these chemicals is reduced or eliminated. Only then can their other food allergies be controlled.

The prevalence of these food chemicals in our modern diet and their potential for provoking illness make it essential that allergic patients be knowledgeable about them. Not understanding their importance, where they hide in the diet, and how to avoid them condemns many patients to a life of pain and discomfort. This is so unnecessary.

TEMPER YOUR DIET WITH COMMON SENSE. Between those patients who follow our dietary advice with religious fervor, never deviating, and those who take a more balanced approach, avoiding the excesses that bring on symptoms—and cheating at times, I find I have much more success with the latter. The former will eventually give up the diet because the strain of unswerving adherence is too great.

The patient who takes a more common-sense approach can stay on the diet for life, if necessary. When cheating causes the return of unpleasant symptoms, it reinforces the need for avoiding the offending food and makes following the diet easier. This patient is also flexible enough to relax his or her vigilance as the need becomes less. For instance, if environmental allergies are treated aggressively with avoidance and allergy injections, the need for total avoidance decreases commensurately. Flexibility and common sense make the diet easier to follow.

DON'T BE DISCOURAGED. It is normal to feel discouraged when asked to eliminate foods and beverages you enjoy— and even crave. It takes awhile to get used to the idea, but our patients tell us that after about three years, they usually forget they are on a diet.

It is often said that success breeds success, and it seems that when the diet has the desired effect of reducing or eliminating our patients' symptoms, it is no longer a burden for them to follow it. When we question our patients about what they eat, we find they have no trouble avoiding the excessive sugar, MSG, low-calorie sweeteners, and acidic foods that once seemed so essential. It can be the same for you.

Adult and Child Allergy Elimination Diet

The diet described in this chapter is given to our patients when they are evaluated in our office and found allergic to food chemicals. It summarizes many of the points discussed in previous chapters.

The purpose of this diet is to help ease the discomfort brought on by reactions to foods. To do this, you must learn which foods and beverages make you ill so that you can avoid them. Food allergy is a common problem, and most of our patients suffer from it to a greater or lesser degree. By learning how to control your food allergy you can reduce its impact on your life.

For the majority of our patients, food allergy reactions result from sensitivity to certain chemicals in our modern diet. Each chemical is made of substances normally present in our bodies and, when consumed in low quantities, does not cause illness. However, today's diet encourages excessive consumption of certain chemicals. If you learn to avoid the foods and beverages that contain high levels these chemicals, you can avoid much pain and discomfort.

The Food Chemicals

The food chemicals that concern us are (1) citric acid, which is commonly found in our diet, and less frequently encountered acids such as malic acid, tartaric acid, fumaric acid, and succinic acid; (2) refined sugar; (3) monosodium glutamate (MSG); and (4) aspartic acid, found in the artificial sweetener aspartame and sold under the brand names Equal® and NutraSweet®. (The artificial sweetener saccharin, sold as Saccharine®, must also be avoided).

Note: Citric acid can also be called citrate or citrus, malic acid can be called malate, tartaric acid can be called tartrate, fumaric acid can be called fumarate, and succinic acid can be called succinate.

The Offending Foods and Beverages

The following foods and beverages contain large quantities of the above chemicals.

THE ACID FOODS AND BEVERAGES. Foods and drinks with high citric and related acids have a citrus or fruity taste. Many are natural—not processed (manufactured). For example, berries, cherries, grapes, and the citrus fruits—oranges, lemons, limes, grapefruit—have naturally high levels of citric acid. Others are processed; a manufacturer will add citric or related acids to a beverage or food to give it a pleasant, fruity taste. This addition is always listed in the ingredients, so watch for the presence of citric acid or less commonly malic, tartaric, fumaric or succinic acid. As mentioned, the acids may also be labeled somewhat differently, with the –ic of citric replaced by –ate, as in sodium or potassium citrate.

If the acid is high on the list of ingredients, the amount in the manufactured food is probably large, so you should avoid eating that product. If the acid is listed toward the end, it is probably present in small amounts and should not bother you. In all cases, let your sense of taste guide you; if it tastes fruity, leave it alone.

The following is a partial list of foods and beverages that contain high amounts of citric acid:

1. Candy, jam, jelly, preserves
2. Carbonated and noncarbonated beverages (soda pop, packaged drink mixes, etc.)
3. Desserts (ice cream, flavored gelatin, pies, puddings, etc.).
4. All fruits and berries listed below:

apricots	grapes	pineapple
blackberries	kiwi	plantains
blue berries	kumquats	plums
cherries	lemons	pomegranates
crab apples	limes	prunes
cranberries	loganberries	raisins
currants	mangos	raspberries
dates	mulberries	rhubarb
figs	nectarines	strawberries
gooseberries	oranges	tangerines
grapefruit		

5. Any fruit juices or juice blends
6. Tomatoes, tomato juice, and tomato-based products
7. All potatoes and potato products (potatoes are acidic)

REFINED SUGAR. Refined sugar is used to sweeten many packaged foods and canned and bottled beverages. It will always be listed on the package, although it is often called by different names: corn syrup, honey, brown sugar, molasses, maple syrup. All are refined sugars and can cause symptoms. You need not pursue a diet completely free of all refined sugar; aim for a diet low enough in refined sugar that your symptoms are not stimulated.

The following is a partial list of foods and beverages high in refined sugar:

1. Candy, jam, jelly, preserves
2. Carbonated and noncarbonated beverages containing sugar
3. Desserts (cakes, cookies, ice cream, flavored gelatin, pies, sweet rolls, presweetened cereals, etc.)

MONOSODIUM GLUTAMATE. High quantities of monosodium glutamate are naturally present in foods such as mushrooms, kelp (seaweed), and scallops. It is commonly used in prepared meats such as breakfast sausages, bratwurst, hot dogs, luncheon meats, pot pies, frozen prepared entrées, and TV dinners. MSG gives these foods an extra hearty taste that is pleasant to the palate but has unpleasant consequences for many allergy sufferers.

Watch for MSG in soups and breaded products, as well as in many snack foods such as crackers, chips, and nuts. It is also used extensively in Chinese cooking, but usually can be avoided by asking the cook to prepare the meal without monosodium glutamate. MSG is released from protein during the fermentation of foods and beverages; therefore, expect to find it in cheese, soy sauce, and alcoholic beverages.

To determine whether processed foods contain MSG, look for it on the label. If you see it listed, do not buy the product. Sometimes MSG is hidden under the catchall phrase "natural flavors"; short of writing to the manufacturer to ask if the "natural flavors" include MSG, there is no way to be sure whether it is present. Even more frequently, it is disguised by being labeled "autolyzed yeast extract" or "hydrolyzed vegetable protein," which contains ten to forty percent MSG. Do not buy such products.

ARTIFICIAL SWEETENERS. Aspartame (NutraSweet® and Equal®) and Saccharine® are commonly found in carbonated and noncarbonated diet beverages, diet foods, and low-calorie sweeteners for home use. My patients must avoid them.

Using the Diet

STARTING OUT. How you start the diet depends on the frequency of your symptoms. It does not matter whether these symptoms are a stuffy nose, headaches, hives, asthma, abdominal pains, diarrhea, or any of the numerous other symptoms that plague the allergic patient. If your symptoms occur frequently—daily or weekly—you will be able to judge the effect of avoiding these chemicals immediately. Meticulously avoid foods and beverages prohibited by the diet for two weeks and watch for improvement in your symptoms.

If your symptoms occur less frequently—monthly or less often—you may not be able to learn anything from two weeks of elimination, even if you follow the diet meticulously. If you were symptom-free, there would be no way to tell if the diet worked or if you simply didn't experience any symptoms during those two weeks. Therefore, you need not completely abstain from these foods and beverages; instead, we ask you to reduce their use to avoid their unpleasant consequences.

If your symptoms appear only during one season or time of the year, you will need to follow this diet during that season only. Seasonal allergy often arouses underlying food allergy that can make you miserable.

DURING THE DIET. If your symptoms are frequent, avoiding the above foods and beverages for a two-week period allows you to determine their effect on your symptoms. If you find them reduced in frequency or severity—fewer or less severe headaches, wheezing, rash, or other illness—these foods are probably at least partly to blame for your symptoms.

If your symptoms are infrequent, you need not follow a strict elimination diet; however, you should be aware of these foods because they may be major causes of your troubles. Avoid eating or drinking excessive amounts. When illness strikes, recall what you have eaten for the previous twenty-four hours; you should be able to identify the offending foods and beverages. They are usually the foods and beverages listed above.

TESTING THE DIET. A second step is necessary to make sure the particular foods and beverages you suspect are actually the cause of your discomfort. Return them to your diet; if your symptoms flare on reintroduction, you will be more confident that they are the cause. How you do it is up to you. It is perfectly acceptable to first reintroduce the foods and beverages you miss the most, adding them back carefully in small quantities or all of them at once in large quantities. Adding one food at a time is probably not helpful; it is the total quantity of all these foods and beverages combined in your diet that causes pain and discomfort.

LIVING WITH THE DIET. As you become accustomed to this diet, you will find that you can eat and drink many of the prohibited foods and beverages if you limit the quantities to a level you can tolerate. For instance, you may be able to eat one or two cookies in a day, but not ten. You may tolerate a little ketchup, but not a glass of tomato juice. You may tolerate some cheese, but probably not as much as you would like. Eventually, you should be able to determine your level of tolerance for these foods and beverages, making the diet less onerous and you more comfortable.

What You Can Eat

A MENU. The following is menu of foods that are generally acceptable for patients who must avoid certain foods and beverages because of sensitivity. To help plan your menu, we listed some name brands of products we believe are low in chemicals that trouble our patients. We regret this is only a partial list; many good products are not listed.

BREAKFAST

Cereals (use any of the following with milk)

Cheerios®	Malt-o-Meal®	Rice Krispies®
Cream of Rice®	Oatmeal®	Shredded Wheat®
Cream of Wheat®	Puffed Rice®	Wheat Chex®
Grapenut Flakes®	Puffed Wheat®	

BREAKFAST cont.

Eggs
Bacon, ham
Toast with butter or margarine

LUNCH

Grain products (may be used at any meal)

Baking powder biscuits	Muffins (banana, bran, free of citric acid and low in sugar)
Breads (rye, wheat, rice)	
Crackers	
Croissants (plain)	Noodles and macaroni
Flat breads	Rice (white rice, wild rice, rice cakes)
Flour tortillas	

The following are lunch suggestions:

- Sandwich with beef, pork, fish or fowl. Butter or margarine are allowed; may be garnished with lettuce or a pickle.

- Salad with oil and vinegar (not wine vinegar), olive oil, or mayonnaise without lemon juice or citrus added. Lettuce, spinach, onion, carrots, cucumbers, radishes, olives, celery. Accompany with any of the allowed fruits.

- Sausage, hamburgers or hot dogs are allowed if free of added MSG, citrus, or other chemicals.

DINNER

Meat—beef, pork, fish, fowl

Salad—same as lunch salad

Grain products—same as for lunch

Vegetables (any of the following):

artichokes	celery
asparagus	okra
beets	olives (without pimento)
boiled broccoli	parsnips
boiled cabbage	radishes
boiled corn	rutabaga
boiled green beans	squash
carrots	turnips

Fruits—you may have two or more servings of:

apples	peaches
bananas	pears
cantaloupe	watermelon
muskmelon	

Beverages

coffee	unflavored bottled water
milk	water
tea	

Snacks—any crackers or pretzels processed without MSG, sugar, or acids; any nuts without additives other than salt: almonds, Brazil nuts, cashews, filberts, hazelnuts, macadamia nuts, pecans, pistachios, sunflower seeds, walnuts.

ACCEPTABLE FOODS BY FOOD GROUP. The following is a partial list of foods that are acceptable for patients on our diet. The foods are classified according to biologic relationship with examples of each group. *If you have a strong allergy to any of these foods (i.e., nuts, fish), you must avoid it—do not use it in the diet.* If you have a weak allergy to some of the foods we list as acceptable, continue to use these foods unless they cause symptoms. Sometimes, eating them one or two days out of three (rotating foods) will allow you to tolerate them.

ANIMAL GROUPS

Amphibians: frogs

Crustaceans: crab, lobster, shrimp

Eggs

Fish: bass, cod, crappie, flounder, haddock, halibut, salmon, scrod, sunfish, trout, tuna, walleye, whitefish

Fowl: chicken, cornish game hen, duck, goose, turkey

Milk products: butter, milk casein (cheese product)

Mollusks: abalone, clams, oysters, snails

Red meat animals: beef, lamb, mutton, pork, veal (roasts, steaks, chops), bacon, ham

PLANT GROUPS

Beech family: beechnut, chestnut

Birch family: filbert, hazelnut

Cashew family: cashew, pistachio

Ginger family: cardamom, ginger

Goosefoot family: beet, spinach, swiss chard

Gourd family: cantaloupe (muskmelon), casaba, cucumber, honeydew melon, pumpkin, squash, watermelon

Grass family: barley, oats, rice, rye, wheat

Laurel family: avocado, bay leaf, cinnamon

Lecythis: Brazil nut

Lily family: asparagus, chives, garlic, leek, onion

Madder family: cottonseed, okra

Mint family: basil, Japanese artichoke, marjoram, mint, oregano, peppermint, sage, savory, spearmint, thyme

Morning glory family: sweet potato, yam

Mustard family: radish, rutabaga, turnip

Myrtle family: allspice

Olive family: olive

Parsley family: caraway, carrot, celeriac, celery, dill, parsley

Pepper family: black pepper

Plum family: almond

Poppy family: poppyseed

Sunflower family: artichoke, Jerusalem artichoke, lettuce, sunflower

Tea family: tea

Walnut family: black walnut, butternut, English hickory nut, pecan

Additional Information

FRUITS. Most of our patients are able to tolerate two or three servings of the recommended fruits, including apples, bananas, cantaloupe, muskmelon, peaches, pears and watermelon. These fruits are lower in acid; avoid the rest.

CHEESE. Many of our patients tolerate only a limited amount of cheese or none at all. Cheese contains MSG; the more aged the cheese, the more MSG it contains.

LEGUMES. Includes beans, peas, peanuts, and soy beans. Sensitivity to these foods varies; you may or may not be able to tolerate them. Storing fresh peas and beans for twenty-four hours before preparing them, boiling them well, and discarding the boiled water helps reduce symptoms in many of our patients.

POTATOES. Potatoes are a special problem. Most of our patients tolerate only a few meals of potatoes per week; others cannot tolerate any potatoes. Use caution and watch your symptoms when you use them in your diet. Boiling them well may be the best way to serve them. Surprisingly, potatoes are closely related to tomatoes.

CORN AND CORN PRODUCTS. Be careful. Corn allergies are common in our patients; perhaps fifty percent react to corn, especially popcorn or corn on the cob. Use caution and watch for symptoms when eating corn products. Cutting corn free from the cob and boiling it well helps many patients tolerate it.

CABBAGE FAMILY. Many patients react poorly to raw cabbage, broccoli, brussel sprouts, and cauliflower but can eat them when boiled until soft.

REFINED SUGAR. Tolerated in small to moderate quantities by many of our patients. If you are moderately sensitive, you should find that honey on bread, a small slice of cake, several cookies, a doughnut or sweet roll, a little pop, or sugar in your coffee can be tolerated. Keep the total amount of refined sugar or honey consumed in a day to a small or moderate quantity.

VINEGAR. Do not use either wine or apple cider vinegar. Use only vinegar made from grain and as small an amount as possible.

VITAMINS AND FOOD SUPPLEMENTS. Stop all vitamins and food supplements during the two-week trial elimination period. Many supplements contain aspartic and glutamic acid (MSG). Vitamin C needs to be combined with citric acid to prevent deterioration.

ALCOHOL. No alcohol should be consumed on the two-week trial elimination.

Dining Out

Dining out is becoming commonplace in our society. For families in which both parents work outside the home, time with the children is too precious to waste on preparing elaborate meals. The health-conscious among us are more apt to spend time jogging or cycling rather than cooking.

Dining out has its advantages—no last-minute shopping, no dishes to wash, no spending time in the kitchen after a hard day at work. Unfortunately, for those of us who suffer debilitating illness from the foods we eat, these advantages are outweighed by one important disadvantage; namely, that we cannot tolerate certain foods restaurants may serve us. However, we can minimize this disadvantage by observing a few rules for dining out.

The first and most obvious rule is to avoid foods you know you are sensitive to. The ones most people react to are tomatoes, potatoes, cheese, and mushrooms (cheese and mushrooms contain high levels of natural MSG). These should, of course, be avoided in any form, including salad dressings and pour-over sauces.

If you are unsure whether an entrée contains any of these foods, you can usually find out simply by asking your waitress or waiter; they often know the ingredients in the meals they serve and can help make your dining experience a pleasant one. In restaurants where the food is cooked to order, cheese or mushrooms may be omitted from many dishes by asking the chef to prepare your meal without them.

The next rule is to be wary of descriptive phrases on the menu such as "special house herbs," "natural seasoning," "our special sauce," or "our special house dressing." These preparations are often made with seasonings that may or may not contain the chemicals restricted on the elimination diet (MSG, citric acid). In these cases, waiters and waitresses may not be reliable sources of information. They may assure you these items do not contain MSG or citric acid even when they do. They are not purposely deceiving you. More than likely, they are unaware of the exact ingredients in these menu items.

A restaurant's staff may not know the exact ingredients of a particular sauce or dressing because they are often prepared from mixes that are manufactured commercially, many of which contain MSG. Much of the information included in this chapter and the next four chapters was gathered by Denise Zang, a member of my staff, and her husband Peter, who is a chef. They tell me they know of only one company, Karlsburger Food Products, that makes sauces and bases for soups and gravies that are free of added MSG. Unfortunately, they only sell their products to the food industry and not to the general public. Since there is no guarantee that a restaurant uses the Karlsburger products I have described, you are better off ordering the item without the sauce or gravy. A safe practice would be to avoid sauces such as hollandaise or bernaise, au jus, gravies, or soups.

Finally, breaded foods are of special concern. MSG is used as a flavor enhancer in prebreaded food products. As a restaurant patron, you have no way of knowing whether the chicken filet you have ordered is prebreaded or if the chef has prepared it himself with fresh bread crumbs. Unless the menu states "fresh bread crumbs," chances are it is a prebreaded item and probably contains MSG.

Over the past few years, Denise has visited many restaurants and talked to managers and chefs about the foods they prepare and serve. She has found that restaurant owners are beginning to recognize the importance of offering tasty, healthy foods, and many of their menu items are now freshly prepared and do not contain added chemicals. A few restaurants even specialize in using only natural ingredients. This change has come about largely because of public pressure; the restaurant business is highly competitive, and this has given the American consumer the power to change the way the industry prepares and serves food.

A good illustration of the public's persuasive power is an experience Denise and her husband Peter had recently at a Chinese restaurant. Like all parents of small children, their evenings out are all too infrequent, so they usually have dinner and see a movie on the same night. On these occasions, Denise prefers Chinese food because she can have a satisfying meal and still have popcorn and pop at the movie a few hours later.

While deciding what to order that evening, Denise noticed a statement written at the bottom of the menu: "Many items are prepared without MSG. Ask your waiter for assistance." Intrigued by this, she asked the hostess if she knew what had prompted the restaurant to offer foods without MSG. The hostess explained that so many people had requested their meals without MSG, the staff decided to prepare as many selections without MSG as with it.

As an experiment, Denise and her husband ordered one item with MSG and one without. They could discern no difference in their meals. Each one tasted as good as the other. Of course, there was one important difference—the one without MSG would not cause Denise the pain and discomfort she normally experiences from this chemical.

The more pressure is brought to bear on restaurant operators, the more change will come about. I must confess that when dining out, I am becoming more comfortable about asking for certain ingredients to be omitted from my meals. Waiters and waitresses are usually very accomodating. The restaurant industry really has nothing to gain by serving the public foods that make them ill.

Quick-Service Restaurants

Not surprisingly, as more and more wives join their husbands in the work force, they find they have less time to spend in the kitchen. The frantic pace of our modern lifestyle has led the busy moms and dads of the world to find other sources of nutritious meals for their families, which has given rise to a burgeoning fast-food industry.

Today there are thousands of quick-service restaurants, many of them part of giant worldwide chains, all trying their best to capture a share of this extremely competitive market. This competition has recently led to changes in the fast-food industry, some of which are favorable for our patients. To attract the health-conscious consumer, many fast-foot chains now feature products that are reduced in fat and cholesterol. A good example is the McLean Deluxe® offered by McDonalds®. It is lower in fat and cholesterol than their regular burgers and is evidence of their conscious effort to respond to health concerns.

The McLean Deluxe® is only one example of this trend. Many fast-foot restaurants have offered salads or salad bars for a number of years, and lately the "burger wars" have given way to "chicken sandwich wars." In addition, the industry is responding to concerns other than fat and cholesterol. Because of heightened awareness about illnesses related to monosodium glutamate, restaurants are now taking great pains to identify and reduce the MSG in their foods. Those of us who are sensitive to foods can now go into just about any quick-service restaurant and find something on the menu to accommodate our dietary requirements, including those of the allergy elimination diet.

To determine which fast foods can be tolerated by patients on the elimination diet, a member of my staff contacted the public relations departments of four quick-service chain restaurants. Their representatives were friendly, helpful, and more than willing to provide us with the information we wanted. Several of them have produced pamphlets or brochures on the nutritional value and content of the foods offered in their franchises. These pamphlets, which are available at the restaurants, include information on serving size, calories, protein, carbohydrate, fat, sodium, and cholesterol content, and a breakdown of the vitamins for each product. They also list the ingredients for each menu item, for instance, lettuce, ground beef, tomatoes, onions, american cheese, citric acid, and MSG.

The willingness of the fast-food industry to respond to dietary restrictions is reflected in other ways as well. You may have heard of Burger King's® advertising campaign to "have it your way," and most quick-service chains encourage comments from their patrons on their products and services. If more of us would question the industry about what goes into their products and make them aware of food and drink ingredients that can cause problems, we would all benefit. No restaurant wants you to get sick from eating their food.

For those who experience debilitating illness from food acids and chemicals like MSG, coping with the everyday problem of trying to grab a bite to eat between picking up the kids up at day care and getting them to ball games or music lessons can be a problem. However, the same rules given in the previous chapter for dining out also pertain to eating at quick-service restaurants, and following them should make it possible to do so without getting sick.

If you are sensitive to tomatoes, you need to be wary of condiments and sauces made with tomatoes such as ketchup and barbecue sauce. Several quick-service restaurants have also invented their "own special sauce" to enhance the flavor of a particular sandwich. These sauces almost always contain MSG, citric acid, or hydrolyzed vegetable protein.

Quick-service sandwiches are frequently garnished with cheese or mushrooms, which are both naturally high in MSG. Some people can tolerate them occasionally, but even they must limit their intake. Remember that foods with breading or coating are also likely to contain MSG.

French fries, hash browns, potato cakes, and potato chips should all be avoided because of their natural citric acid content. Finally, stay away from any item that is high in sugar—pastries, pies, ice cream, cheesecake, and cookies. Soft-serve yogurt also contains sugar, in addition to MSG.

To illustrate how easy it is to make good meal choices at quick-service restaurants, let's spend a busy Saturday with one of my patients and eat at a different one for each meal. She hasn't had time to grocery shop during the week and there's not enough cereal to go around; ballet lessons are at ten o'clock, so let's stop at Burger King® for breakfast. That way we can go to McDonalds® for lunch so her four-year-old can get a Happy Meal® with a surprise inside.

Let's start by ordering french toast sticks. They make a great breakfast for the little ones; toddlers like nothing better than feeding themselves, and the french toast sticks and milk are easy for them to eat. If you tolerate sugar, you can have a tiny bit of syrup. Too much hides the taste of the french toast. It you are sensitive to sugar, the french toast still tastes great without the syrup.

Eggs and toast are alternative choices that are also acceptable on the elimination diet. Maybe you can have both! If you're like most of us, you'll need a cup of coffee to start the morning off right. Cream is okay, but forget the sugar.

After the lessons, there's just enough time to get gas for the car and pick up the dry cleaning before lunch. Dad's softball tournament starts at one o'clock, so let't head for the "golden arches."

There are several choices for lunch at McDonalds® that are acceptable on the elimination diet. Just keep the rules in mind when making your selection. For instance, if you choose a quarter pounder, order it without the cheese or ketchup. (If your children have food allergies, don't forget to order their Happy Meals® the same way.) Or how about a garden salad without the tomato or cheese? A McLean Deluxe® is another option, but with three changes—no tomato, no cheese, and no ketchup. Another cup of coffee sounds good, and let's order milk for the kids.

After the softball game, there's just enough time to do the grocery shopping and get everything put away before it's off to Wendy's® for dinner. Let's start off with a salad because the salad bar at Wendy's® offers many of the fruits and vegetables permitted on the diet—lettuce, bananas, chunky apple sauce, three-bean salad, watermelon, honeydew melon, chives, carrots, cantaloupe, or alfalfa sprouts. We can also have a grilled chicken sandwich; Wendy's® makes one without breading. It is topped with a honey-mustard sauce, but we'll ask them to leave it off. This time let's order milk; too much coffee can keep you awake at night.

There, we did it. A whole day of running errands, chauffeuring kids, and eating out. We got a lot accomplished and kept the whole family fed and happy.

Grazing

Most of us are so busy with our daily lives—school, jobs, family—we have little time for regular, planned meals. Instead we rush from school to work or from errand to errand, grabbing a snack as time permits. This form of eating is popularly referred to as "grazing."

Webster's Dictionary defines *grazing* as:

> **1.** To feed on growing grass and pasturage, as do cattle, sheep, etc. **2.** To eat small portions of food, as appetizers or the like, in place of a full-sized meal or to snack during the course of the day in place of regular meals. **3.** To feed on (growing grass).

Eating frequent small meals on the run makes it difficult to be selective about what is included in these meals. For some, grazing is a daily habit and often leads to illness, most likely because they consume too much of foods they do not tolerate well—foods such as citrus fruits, some raw vegetables, candy, cookies, cakes, potato chips, pop, acidic foods, low-calorie sweeteners, and foods that contain refined sugar or MSG.

Having to avoid foods and beverages you enjoy can be discouraging, and it can be even more discouraging if it means making big changes in your lifestyle. But there are several ways to reduce the complexity involved in following the elimination diet, and it is even possible to graze and still satify hunger if foods and beverages that cause illness are avoided. Here are a few simple tips to help you do that.

Weekends are a busy time for most families. There are errands to run and chores to do, which leaves little or no time for organized meals. This can be a problem, especially if you have children, who think they need to eat every half hour. I'm sure most of you are familiar with phrases like "I'm hungry" or "I'm thirsty" and the question that seems to be asked most often, "What can I have to eat?"

With a little planning and preparation, you can provide quick meals and snacks using foods that are tolerated on the elimination diet. For instance, apples, cantaloupe, pears, muskmelon, peaches, bananas, and watermelon are all acceptable, which is quite a list of fruits. It's a good idea to keep two or three different types on hand at all times.

Many vegetables are also acceptable, including carrots, celery, cucumbers, olives, radishes, beets, squash, asparagus, okra, artichokes, rutabagas, and turnips. They are usually well tolerated by people with food-related illness.

Preparation of these fruits and vegetables does not have to be a horrendous task. Take a few minutes as soon as you get home from shopping to wash fruits such as apples, peaches, and pears. The Food and Drug Administration recommends thoroughly washing fruits and vegetables to remove any chemical residues. Foods such as melons, carrots, celery, and cucumbers can be quickly cleaned, cut up, and stored in the refrigerator in plastic containers or locking storage bags. Nutritious fruits and vegetables can be handed out as easily as sticks of gum or candy, or children can help themselves (within reason) when they get the urge to graze. Eating a banana or a carrot stick is as easy as eating a candy bar. Which one children select depends on which one is most accessible to them.

Crackers are a good accompaniment with light meals, and there are many wholesome varieties available today. Label reading is very important when buying crackers because ingredients vary from manufacturer to manufacturer. By carefully checking the labels, you can determine which are most likely to be tolerated. Avoid ingredients like MSG and hydrolyzed vegetable protein; both have the potential to cause problems.

Once you have figured out which brands are tolerated, keep plenty on hand. When serving a sandwich, fill the plate with a handful of crackers instead of potato chips and then add any of the fruits and vegetables listed in this chapter. This combination is great for lunch boxes too.

Slicing fruits and vegetables and placing them on crackers makes a tasty snack, and children think it is great fun to eat finger foods. Little sandwiches made with crackers are also a nice change from bread and are much crunchier! Those who study the psychological effects of eating report that crunchier foods are a lot more satisfying.

If you tolerate peanut butter, it goes great with crackers or bread. You can also make a great snack by spreading peanut butter on a celery stick.

Avoiding the beverages prohibited by the elimination diet often seems to pose a difficult problem. Our modern lifestyle relies heavily on the sweet or fruity drinks, both carbonated and noncarbonated, that come in convenient cans or bottle, but many of them contain citric or other food acids or are made from the juices of prohibited fruits. A number of beverages are allowed, however, and are usually just as satisfying.

Of course, the first beverage that comes to mind is the one Mother Nature provides for us. Water is essential to our lives because it is part of every important process that takes place in our bodies. Many doctors stress the value of drinking four to six glasses of water a day, especially for dieters and pregnant women.

Get into the habit of keeping a pitcher of water in the refrigerator at all times. Ice cold water is thirst quenching and good for you. What's more, it's available everywhere.

Aside from water, coffee is probably the most frequently consumed beverage. Many of us drink coffee from morning until night. For a change of pace on hot days, why not try iced coffee? After brewing the coffee, pour it into a pitcher, add ice cubes, and refrigerate it. In a short time, you'll have a refreshing summer cooler, a definite improvement over the citrus-filled carbonated beverages that cause many of us distress.

Tea is another beverage that can be enjoyed hot or cold, and a number of instant iced tea products are available today. Although many contain citric acid, there are a few that do not. Lipton® makes an iced tea with no sugar or lemon that is a good one to try. Check the labels on other products carefully before using them.

Nature provides us with another drink, one that Denise and Peter Zang fondly refer to as the "Holstein Highball." As the name *holstein* implies, it is the drink derived from the animal better known as the cow.

Milk is often thought of as the perfect food for babies and adults alike, but for some people, it is not the answer. It can cause diarrhea, pain, and discomfort. Watch your own symptoms and let your body's reaction be your guide.

I hope these ideas reassure you that it is possible to follow the elimination diet with very little effect on your style of living. With a little preplanning, label reading, and getting rid of troublesome food items from your kitchen, you will be able to graze safely and avoid the distressing symptoms brought on by eating too many foods you aren't able to tolerate.

Shopping

In the 1800s, before the advent of the commercial food processing industry, women and men knew the contents of their foods because they planted, harvested, milled, and canned the grains, fruits, and vegetables themselves. Beef, pork, and poultry were raised on the family farm and then slaughtered when reserves became low. The food was free of added chemicals such as preservatives or flavor enhancers.

While the early settlers did not have to worry about chemicals in their foods, they also did not have the luxury of running to the corner market when they needed a loaf of bread, milk, or meat. Preparing the evening meal often took the entire day. For example, if a loaf of bread was needed, they had to cut the wheat, grind it into flour, mix the flour with eggs, milk, and sugar, and let it rise all day before baking it over an open hearth.

Fortunately, we don't have to go through the same processes as the women and men of the 1800s to provide our families with nutritious meals. Instead we can go to the supermarket and buy our foods and beverages, many of them already prepared. However, we are faced with the growing problem of food additives—citric, malic, and fumaric acids, monosodium glutamate, hydrolyzed vegetable protein, refined sugar, and low-calorie sweeteners.

As consumers of prepared food products, how can we make it easier to select foods and beverages that are allowed on the elimination diet and avoid the harmful foods and food additives? We are familiar with the list of foods and beverages that are not acceptable when following the diet; tomatoes, potatoes, cheese, citrus fruits, and pop are easily recognized and avoided while doing the weekly grocery shopping. The more difficult ingredients to identify are the chemicals and additives found in these foods.

One way to identify them is by becoming knowledgeable label readers. The Food and Drug Administration (FDA) helps us do this by requiring food and beverage processors to label their products not only with nutritional values, but also with specific ingredients found in the foods. However, ingredient labels can still be misleading. For instance, hydrolyzed vegetable protein, which contains MSG, is poorly tolerated by many who follow the elimination diet. This additive should not be confused with hydrogenated oils, which are usually tolerated. *Natural flavors* is another term sometimes used to describe MSG. Describing MSG as *natural* is factual because it is found naturally in many foods.

To illustrate the various terms food processors use, the lists of ingredients for several types of prepackaged foods are reproduced in this chapter. When the list of ingredients contains chemicals that are poorly tolerated by my patients, they are highlighted to call your attention to them. Avoid eating foods with these ingredients. If no ingredients are highlighted, the foods are acceptable for patients with food allergy.

As mentioned earlier, certain chemicals such as sugar and the fruit acids are well tolerated if present in small quantities. When they are present in small quantities, the foods will not have a strong sweet or fruity taste and the sugar or acid will be listed near the end of the list of ingredients. Foods containing MSG, low-calorie sweeteners, or pronounced sweet or fruity flavors must be avoided.

Spaghetti Noodles

INGREDIENTS: SEMOLINA, NIACINAMIDE, FERROUS SULFATE (IRON), THIAMINE MONONITRATE AND RIBOFLAVIN.

Note: Contains no problem ingredients.

Complete Buttermilk Pancake Mix

INGREDIENTS: BLEACHED ENRICHED FLOUR [(BLEACHED FLOUR, MALTED BARLEY FLOUR, NIACIN, IRON, THIAMINE, MONONITRATE (VITAMIN B1), RIBOFLAVIN (VITAMIN B2)], YELLOW CORN FLOUR, **SUGAR**, **DEXTROSE**, BAKING POWDER (BAKING SODA, MONOCALCIUM PHOSPHATE, SODIUM ALUMINUM PHOSPHATE), BUTTERMILK, SALT, EGG WHITES, MONO AND DIGLYCERIDES, NONFAT MILK, LECITHIN, EGGS, HYDROGENATED SOYBEAN OIL, **CORN SYRUP SOLIDS**.

The various forms of sugar have been highlighted in the above ingredient list. Refined sugar can be a problem for many people if it is consumed in too large a quantity. Unfortunately, the Food and Drug Administration does not require food processors to include on the label what percentage of the total product content is accounted for by a particular ingredient. Instead, ingredients are listed in descending order of content, with the ingredient accounting for the highest percentage of the total product listed first.

In the pancake mix above, sugar is the third ingredient, listed, dextrose is the fourth, and another form of sugar—corn syrup solids—ends the list. Although the label does not tell us what percentage of the total content these sugars represent, this mix probably contains too much sugar for patients on our diet. If the item tastes sweet, you should not eat it; no matter where it is listed in the ingredient list, the sugar content is probably too high.

Skillet Hamburger Mix

> INGREDIENTS: ENRICHED MACARONI, VEGETABLE SHORT-ENING (CONTAINS ONE OR BOTH OF THE FOLLOWING PARTIALLY HYDROGENATED OILS: SOYBEAN, COTTONSEED), **CHEDDAR CHEESE**, (MILK, SALT, CHEESE CULTURES, ENZYMES, COLOR ADDED), CORN STARCH, **TOMATO** (WITH COLOR PROTECTED BY SODIUM BISULFITE), BUTTERMILK, SALT, **SUGAR**, **HYDROLYZED VEGETABLE PROTEIN**, ONION, **CORN SYRUP**, DISODIUM PHOSPHATE (FOR SMOOTH SAUCE), GARLIC, NATURAL FLAVORS, SODIUM CASEINATE (A MILK PROTEIN), **CITRIC ACID**, (FOR FLAVOR), DIPOTASSIUM PHOSPHATE (FOR SMOOTH SAUCE), YELLOW 5 AND YELLOW 6.

Note: Don't use this mix.

Chicken Coating Mix

> INGREDIENTS: BLEACHED BROMATED WHEAT FLOUR, **DEXTRIN** (FROM CORN), PARTIALLY HYDROGENATED SOYBEAN AND COTTONSEED OILS, SALT, PAPRIKA, MALTED BARLEY, SPICES (MUSTARD FLOUR, CELERY SEED, CHILI PEPPER, BLACK PEPPER, THYME, BASIL, RED PEPPER, CLOVES, OREGANO, ROSEMARY), **SUGAR**, YEAST, BEET POWDER (FOR COLOR), GARLIC POWDER, ONION POWDER, NATURAL HICKORY SMOKE FLAVOR, TBHQ AND CALCIUM PROPIO-NATE (TO PRESERVE FRESHNESS).

This coating mix does not contain MSG or hydrolyzed vegetable protein, but it does contain sugars. If you use it, you may experience discomfort, especially if other poorly tolerated foods are consumed in the same time period.

Canned Meat

> INGREDIENTS: CHOPPED PORK SHOULDER MEAT WITH HAM MEAT ADDED AND SALT, WATER, SUGAR, SODIUM NITRATE.

Chicken Flavor Rice Mix

INGREDIENTS: ENRICHED EGG WHITE MACARONI PROD-
UCT, NATURAL FLAVORS, SALT, PARTIALLY HYDROGENATED
VEGETABLE OIL (SOYBEAN AND OR COTTONSEED), FOOD
STARCH, **MODIFIED CORN SYRUP, SUGAR**, CHICKEN,
MONOSODIUM GLUTAMATE, ONIONS, MODIFIED VEGE-
TABLE GUM, SODIUM CASEINATE, GARLIC, YEAST, CHICKEN
BROTH, SOY FLOUR, PARSLEY, SPICE, DISODIUM INOSINATE,
DISODIUM GUANYLATE.

Because this mix contains MSG (monosodium glutamate) as well as sugars, avoid using it. The combination of
these chemicals is likely to cause problems. Note that the
term "natural flavors" is also listed. There is no way of
knowing whether this term includes MSG, but I believe
that most food processors do not use MSG without men-
tioning it on the label. Therefore, it is not necessary to avoid
a product because it contains natural flavors. Assume that
the product is acceptable and hope for the best.

Gelatin Dessert

INGREDIENTS: **SUGAR**, GELATIN, ADIPIC ACID (FOR TART-
NESS), DISODIUM PHOSPHATE (CONTROLS ACIDITY),
FUMARIC ACID (FOR TARTNESS), ARTIFICIAL COLOR, ARTI-
FICIAL FLAVOR.

Note: This product is probably too sweet.

Instant Pudding

INGREDIENTS: **SUGAR, DEXTROSE (CORN SUGAR)**, CORN
STARCH MODIFIED, SODIUM PHOSPHATES (FOR PROPER
SET), SALT, HYDROGENATED SOYBEAN OIL WITH BHA
(PRESERVATIVE), DI AND MONOGLYCERIDES (PREVENT
FOAMING), NONFAT MILK, ARTIFICIAL COLOR (INCLUDING
YELLOW 5 AND YELLOW 6), ARTIFICIAL AND NATURAL
FLAVOR.

Note: Contains too much sugar.

Tuna in Spring Water

INGREDIENTS: CHUNK LIGHT TUNA IN SPRING WATER, VEGETABLE BROTH, SALT, **HYDROLYZED PROTEIN.**

Note: Don't use this product.

Fruit Juice

INGREDIENTS: **GRAPE, APPLE AND PASSION FRUIT JUICES,** FROM CONCENTRATES, NATURAL FLAVOR, VITAMIN C.

Note: This product is probably too acidic; don't use it.

Pear Halves in Heavy Syrup

INGREDIENTS: PEARS, WATER, **CORN SYRUP** AND **SUGAR.**

Note: May be used if syrup is rinsed off thoroughly.

Label reading is a skill developed over time. If you eat or drink something that causes you to experience symptoms, check the label; the product may contain an item not acceptable on the elimination diet. As you learn to recognize the problematic food additives and chemicals by name, it will be easier to avoid buying products that contain them.

Recipes

Have you ever wondered what to do on a rainy Saturday afternoon after the laundry's done, the house cleaned, the closets rearranged, the dog bathed, the garage swept, the bathroom retiled, the entire house repainted? How about preparing a nice meal. Denise and Peter Zang have collected a number of recipes ranging from easy to difficult. To the best of our knowledge, they are tolerated while observing the restrictions of the elimination diet. If you are sensitive to any of the foods or ingredients mentioned, find another recipe that does not include this food or ingredient.

You will notice that many of the recipes contain sugar or honey. Most of our patients tolerate limited amounts of sugar and honey, and we tried to minimize the use of both while preserving some of the sweetness.

Easy Recipes

BROILED CHICKEN

Chickens weighing 2½ pounds or less are good for broiling. Cut the whole chicken into halves or quarters. Turn wing tips to back side. Place chicken, skin side down, on rack in broiler pan. Brush chicken with melted margarine or butter and a little garlic. Place broiler pan so top of chicken is 7 to 9 inches from heat. Broil chicken 30 minutes. Sprinkle brown side with salt and pepper as desired. Turn chicken; brush with melted margarine. Broil until chicken is crisp and brown and thickest pieces are done, 20 to 30 minutes longer.

CHICKEN CHANGES

Dip chicken or pork chops in an egg wash of slightly beaten eggs and milk and then in crushed dry cereal such as Special K®, Wheaties®, Product 19® or Total®. Pan fry or bake at 350°. This is a new and easy way to enjoy chicken or pork chops.

CHICKEN WITH GARLIC

3- to 4-pound roasting chicken
2 pounds garlic cloves

Preheat oven to 350°. Rinse chicken under cold water, inside and out, and pat dry with paper towels. Peel the cloves of garlic and arrange them in the center at the bottom of a roasting pan. Place the chicken on the bed of garlic cloves and bake for 1 to 1¼ hours, basting from time to time during the last 30 minutes. Season to taste. Serves 4.

EASY OVEN-FRIED CHICKEN

1 whole chicken cut into 8 pieces, or a package of chicken
   parts you prefer
¾ cup cornmeal
Corn oil
½ teaspoon garlic powder
Salt and pepper to taste

Preheat oven to 350°. Wash and pat the chicken dry with a paper towel. Place the cornmeal, seasonings, and chicken in a strong plastic or paper bag. Close securely and shake until the chicken is well coated. Brush or pour a thin layer of oil in the baking pan. Place the coated chicken parts on the oiled pan. Bake for 1 hour, turning once in the course of baking.

Medium Difficulty Recipes

HAM-IT-UP SNACKS

8-ounce package Pillsbury Crescent Rolls®
4 thin slices ham (or more)
4 teaspoons mustard
4 ounces (1 cup) imitation low-moisture, part skim
    mozzarella cheese
2 tablespoons sesame seeds

Heat oven to 375°. Unroll dough into four long rectangles. Press perforations to seal. Lay ham on dough. Spread ham with mustard and sprinkle with cheese. Starting at shortest side, roll up each rectangle, seal edges, and coat rolls with sesame seeds. Cut each roll into five slices, forming 20 slices in all. Place cut side down on ungreased cookie sheet. Bake at 375° for 15 to 20 minutes until golden brown. Serve.

Note: Imitation cheese may bother some patients.

CROUTONS

5 slices day-old white or wheat bread
3 tablespoons butter or margarine
½ teaspoon garlic powder
½ teaspoon onion salt

Cut bread into cubes. Melt butter and add garlic powder and onion salt. Pour over bread cubes; mix well. Spread cubes on a cookie sheet and bake in 350° oven until golden brown. This is a great addition to any salad.

A Few Words about Salads

When preparing a fresh lettuce salad, remember it doesn't necessarily have to be made with iceberg lettuce. Instead try using one or a combination of the following types: bibb lettuce, Boston red leaf lettuce, curly endive, endive, escarole, leaf lettuce, romaine, spinach, or watercress. They can be found at most larger grocery stores. They will not only give your salad a different taste but a different look as well.

For toppings, try one or more of the following: ripe olives, bacon bits (fry or microwave until crisp, break into bits, and store in bowl in freezer until ready to use), sunflower seeds, sliced onion, sliced turkey, chicken, etc.

BUTTERMILK DRESSING

¾ cup Miracle Whip®
½ cup buttermilk
1 teaspoon parsley flakes
½ teaspoon minced onion (instant)
1 clove garlic, crushed
½ teaspoon salt
Pinch ground pepper

Shake well and refrigerate.

HERB DRESSING

⅓ cup olive oil or vegetable oil
3 tablespoons grain-based vinegar
1 teaspoon salt
1 teaspoon dried tarragon leaves
¼ teaspoon dried basil leaves
1 large clove garlic, crushed

Shake all ingredients in tightly covered jar and refrigerate.

ITALIAN DRESSING

1 cup vegetable oil
¼ cup grain-based vinegar
1 teaspoon salt
1 teaspoon sugar
½ teaspoon dry mustard
½ teaspoon onion salt
½ teaspoon paprika
½ teaspoon dry oregano leaves
⅛ teaspoon ground thyme leaves
2 cloves garlic, crushed

Shake ingredients in tightly covered jar and refrigerate at least 2 hours. Shake before serving.

PORKBURGERS

For a change of pace from that plain old hamburger, use ground pork instead. Add onions, salt and pepper, garlic, oregano, and basil for seasonings. Form into patties and fry in a pan, broil, or grill on the barbecue. Serve on a bun topped with crispy lettuce.

HOT DOG ROLLUPS

For a quick afternoon lunch or evening supper, try Hot Dog Rollups. Be sure to use hot dogs that don't contain MSG. Wrap buttered white bread corner-to-corner around the hot dog and secure with a toothpick. Bake in 350° oven until the bread turns golden brown.

EGG IN A BASKET

Sunday is family breakfast day—the one day of the week we all sit down to breakfast together. Egg in a Basket is a different way to serve eggs and toast.

In a fry pan, melt a pat of butter or margarine. While it is melting, use a glass to cut a hole in the middle of a piece of white or wheat bread. Place the bread with the hole in it in the fry pan. Crack an egg into the hole and cook until the egg is set. When the bread is brown on one side, turn it over and brown the other side. The egg cooks at the same time.

You can make the egg any way you like—sunny side up, over easy, over hard, scrambled.

BREAD DUMPLINGS

6 slices of bread (cut up)
¼ cup onion (sautéed)
½ cup milk
2 eggs
3 sprigs fresh parsley (chopped)

Combine all ingredients in a bowl until the mixture binds. Form into balls. Refrigerate until ready to use. To cook, boil in salted water 8 to 10 minutes. A good substitute for potatoes.

CARROT SALAD

6 carrots
½ to ¾ cup unflavored yogurt (if you tolerate yogurt)
1 tablespoon honey (if you tolerate honey)
¾ teaspoon ground cinnamon
Pinch of salt

Pare the carrots and grate in a processor or on a grater, using the coarse side. Add the yogurt, honey, cinnamon, and salt. Mix well and chill before serving. Makes two generous servings.

BEEF STOCK

1 quart water
2 to 3 carrots
3 celery stalks
1 small onion
2 bay leaves
1 to 1½ pounds beef scraps (bones, shanks)
Salt and pepper to taste

Boil all ingredients for 1 to 1½ hours; strain broth and discard vegetables and meat. Keeps in refrigerator for four to seven days.

CHICKEN STOCK

1 quart water
2 to 3 carrots
3 celery stalks
1 small onion
1 bay leaf
1 to 2 pounds chicken pieces (backs, necks, wings)
Salt and pepper to taste

Boil all ingredients for 1 to 1½ hours; strain broth and discard vegetables and meat. Keeps in refrigerator for four to seven days.

CABBAGE SOUP

3 tablespoons butter
½ small head green cabbage, thinly sliced (if tolerated)
4 cups beef or chicken stock
1 clove garlic, peeled and minced

1 teaspoon dried dillweed
½ teaspoon dried thyme
Salt and pepper
Optional: 2 tablespoons yogurt (if tolerated)

In a 2-quart saucepan, heat the butter with the seasonings. Add the cabbage and sauté over medium-high heat, stirring often, until the volume reduces and the cabbage begins to brown (a few minutes). Add the stock and bring to a boil. Lower the head and cover, stirring from time to time. Cook 10 minutes. Serves 4.

For French Onion soup, use four large onions, sliced thinly, instead of the cabbage and omit the dill and thyme. Garnish the soup with toast or croutons (see recipe on p. 137).

COLD CUCUMBER SOUP

2 cucumbers
2 scallions
1 cup yogurt (if you tolerate yogurt)
¼ teaspoon powdered cumin
¼ teaspoon garlic powder
Salt and pepper

Peel the cucumbers and cut into 2-in. segments. Wash and trim the scallions and cut them into 2-inch lengths. Place all the ingredients and seasonings in the blender and blend thoroughly. Chill the soup thoroughly (3 to 4 hours) before serving. Serves 2.

LIVER DUMPLING SOUP

½ pound beef liver
4 to 6 slices bread (cut into small pieces)
1 ½ tablespoons butter
2 tablespoons minced onion
1 egg
½ teaspoon marjoram
Salt and pepper to taste
Beef stock

Sauté onion in butter. Mix all ingredients together, adding bread a little at a time so dumpling mixture binds; form into balls and cook in beef stock 15 minutes. Serve in bowl with chopped parsley.

TURKEY VEGETABLE SOUP

Turkey carcass
2 to 4 stalks celery
1 small onion
3 medium carrots
1 small rutabaga
1 small bunch fresh parsley

Break apart turkey and place in Dutch oven. Cover with water and bring to boil. Reduce heat; simmer for 1 hour. Remove from heat, cool, and remove bones. Cut up remaining ingredients and add to stock and meat. Return to heat and simmer until vegetables are tender. Salt and pepper to taste.

Don't forget to use up some of those leftover vegetables and turkey. What a better place than soup!

BAKED HONEY-CINNAMON APPLES

Core baking apples (Rome, Beauty, Golden Delicious) and pare a 1-in. strip of skin from around the middle of each apple to prevent splitting. Place apples upright in ungreased baking dish. Place 1 teaspoon honey, 1 teaspoon margarine or butter, and ⅛ teaspoon ground cinnamon in the center of each apple and pour water ¼ inch deep into baking dish. Bake apples uncovered at 375° until tender when pierced with a fork, about 30 to 40 minutes. Time will vary with the size of the apples. Spoon syrup in dish over apples several times during baking, if desired.

Note: Honey is a refined sugar, and this recipe may contain too much for you.

HOT SPICED PEARS

8 canned pear halves without juice
1 cup water
1 cinnamon stick
4 cloves
⅛ teaspoon nutmeg
1 tablespoon plus 1 teaspoon cornstarch, dissolved in
   1 tablespoon water
1 teaspoon honey

In medium saucepan, combine first five ingredients. Simmer for 5 minutes, stirring constantly; add cornstarch and cook until slightly thickened. Remove and discard cinnamon stick and cloves. Stir in honey. Serve in dessert dishes.

BATTER FOR DEEP FRYING

1 cup flour
¼ teaspoon salt
3 tablespoons olive oil or cooled, melted butter
1 cup water
2 eggs, separated

Mix together the flour, salt, and oil or butter in a bowl. Gradually add the water and whisk for only as long as it takes to produce a smooth batter. Whisk in the egg yolks, but do not overwork the mixture. Leave the batter to rest for at least 1 hour at room temperature; otherwise it will shrink away from the vegetable pieces and provide an uneven coating. Beat the egg whites until they form soft peaks and fold them into the batter just before using it.

Note: This recipe will work for any of the raw vegetables permitted on the elimination diet. It is also great for coating fish, meats, or poultry.

DILL SAUCE

2 tablespoons butter
1 tablespoon onion (chopped fine)
1 teaspoon parsley (chopped)
3 tablespoons flour
1 cup chicken stock or water
Salt and pepper to taste
3 tablespoons dill (chopped)
4 cups plain yogurt

Heat butter in a sauce pan. Add onion and parsley. Sauté for 1 minute. Add flour, cook for 2 minutes. Do not brown. Add broth. Blend and simmer for 5 minutes until smooth and thick. Add all other ingredients. Blend and simmer for 5 minutes. Serve over warm vegetables.

Note: This recipe contains a large amount of yogurt, which may bother some patients.

CRISPY BREAD STICKS

1 cup whole wheat flour
1 package active dry yeast
½ tablespoon sugar
1 teaspoon salt
⅔ cup hot water
2 tablespoons vegetable oil
1 to 1 ¼ cups all-purpose flour

Stir together whole wheat flour, yeast, sugar, and salt. Blend in water and oil and beat until smooth. Stir in enough flour to form soft dough; turn onto a floured surface and continue to work in flour until dough is stiff enough to knead. Knead until smooth and elastic (about 5 minutes), working in as much flour as possible (the more flour, the crispier the bread sticks). Cover and let rest 30 minutes. Divide dough into quarters. Divide each quarter into eight equal pieces. Allow dough to rest 10 minutes; then roll each piece into 10-in. lengths with palms of hand. Place on greased baking sheets about ½ inch apart. If desired, brush with mixture of 1 egg white and 1 teaspoon water. Bake at 325° for 20 minutes. Makes 32 bread sticks.

RICE MEDLEY

1 17-ounce can peas and tiny onions, drained and rinsed
1 ½ cups uncooked instance rice (without MSG)
1 teaspoon butter
½ teaspoon salt
1 small carrot, shredded

Pour 1 ½ cups water into 2-quart sauce pan. Heat to boiling; stir in peas, rice, butter, salt, and carrot. Heat to boiling again. Remove from heat; cover and let stand until all liquid is absorbed and rice is tender, about 10 minutes.

BEEF AND BROWN RICE

1 teaspoon oil
2 medium onions
¾ pound ground beef
2 cups cooked brown rice
1 clove garlic, peeled and minced
Salt and pepper

Heat the oil in a skillet. Peel and chop the onions (if you use scallions, wash and pat dry before cutting). Sauté the onions over medium-high heat for 7 to 10 minutes until golden. Add the meat and sauté, stirring occasionally to keep both onions and meat from burning. Add the garlic, salt, and pepper. Reduce heat and cover. Combine the brown rice with the contents of the skillet, preferably in an attractive bowl, and mix together. Serves 2 generously.

BEEF STEAKS AND CARROTS

⅓ cup all-purpose flour
½ teaspoon salt
⅛ teaspoon pepper
4 beef cubed steaks (about 4 ounces each)
2 tablespoons vegetable oil
1 jar (16-ounce) whole baby carrots, drained
1 envelope Lipton Onion Soup Mix, mixed with 10
    ounces water
½ teaspoon parsley flakes
⅛ teaspoon dried rosemary leaves, crushed

Mix flour, salt, and pepper; coat beef with flour mixture. Heat oil over medium-high heat until hot. Cook beef in oil until brown, about 4 minutes on each side (add more oil if necessary). Stir in remaining ingredients. Heat to boiling; reduce heat. Simmer uncovered until carrots are hot, about 5 minutes.

GARLIC CRUNCH CHICKEN

1¼ pounds boneless chicken parts, skin removed
1 tablespoon plus 1 teaspoon reduced-calorie Miracle
    Whip®
¾ ounce bran cereal flakes, slightly crushed
⅛ teaspoon garlic powder
Salt and pepper to taste
2 teaspoons vegetable oil
1 teaspoon honey

Preheat oven to 350°. Place chicken in a shallow baking pan sprayed with a nonstick cooking spray. Spread Miracle Whip® evenly over top side of chicken. Sprinkle cereal crumbs evenly over chicken. Then sprinkle with garlic powder, salt, and pepper. Drizzle oil and honey evenly over chicken. Bake 30 minutes, uncovered.

HOT BEEF SANDWICHES

4 pounds beef tip or rolled rump roast
2 tablespoons vegetable oil
3 cups beef stock
1 medium onion, cut into fourths
2 cloves garlic, crushed
1 teaspoon pepper
¾ cup cold water
⅓ cup flour
6 hamburger buns, split

Cook beef in oil over medium heat in Dutch oven until brown. Add beef stock, onion, garlic, and pepper. Heat to boiling. Reduce heat; cover and simmer until beef is tender, about 3 hours. Remove beef from broth and shred into small pieces. Strain broth and add enough water to measure 4 cups. Skim excess fat; heat to boiling. Shake flour and water in container as you would for gravy. Add to broth, stirring constantly. Boil and then add shredded beef. When you serve the sandwiches, pile the beef on a bun and cover with gravy

This recipe makes enough for two meals, so you can freeze some for later.

LONDON BROIL

1 to 1½ pounds high-quality beef flank steak
2 medium onions (sliced thin)
¼ teaspoon salt
1 tablespoon butter
2 tablespoons vegetable oil
2 cloves garlic (crushed)
½ teaspoon salt
¼ teaspoon pepper

Cut both sides of beef with diamond pattern, ⅛ in. deep. Cook onions in ¼ teaspoon salt and butter until tender (keep warm). Mix remaining ingredients and brush beef with half of the mixture. Set oven control to broil or 550° on your charcoal grill. Broil beef 2 to 3 inches from heat until brown, about 5 minutes. Turn beef, brush with remaining oil mixture, and broil 5 minutes longer. Thinly slice beef at an angle across the grain; serve with onions. Flank steak, which is not very tender, does not usually broil well, but it when cooked rare and cut thinly across the grain, it's delicious.

SWISS STEAK

3 tablespoons all-purpose flour
1 teaspoon dry mustard
½ teaspoon salt
1½ pounds beef boneless bottom or top round
2 tablespoons vegetable oil
1 large onion

Mix flour, mustard, and salt. Sprinkle one side of beef with half the flour mixture; pound in. Cut beef into six pieces. Heat oil in 10-inch skillet until hot. Cover beef with sliced onion and cook over medium heat until brown, about 15 minutes. Add enough water to cover and cook until beef is tender, about one hour.

SALMON LOAF

1-pound can salmon
2 tablespoons butter
¼ cup cracker crumbs
2 eggs, beaten slightly
¼ cup milk
½ cup parsley flakes
Dash of salt and pepper
½ cup chopped celery

Mix together, put in buttered pan, and set in pan of water. Bake 30 minutes at 350°.

SAUCE
Liquid from salmon
1 tablespoon butter
1 cup milk

Heat; pour over salmon and serve. Grated carrots can be added to salmon mixture.

SWEET POTATO BISCUITS

1¼ cup all-purpose flour
1 tablespoon baking powder
1 teaspoon brown sugar

½ teaspoon salt
⅓ cup shortening
1 beaten egg
½ cup mashed cooked sweet potato
2 tablespoons milk

In mixing bowl, stir together the flour, baking powder, brown sugar, and salt. Cut in shortening until mixture resembles coarse crumbs. Combine egg, mashed sweet potato, and milk; add all at once to dry mixture. Stir just until dough clings together. Knead gently on lightly floured surface (10 to 12 minutes). Roll or pat dough to ½-inch thickness. Cut with a 2½-inch biscuit cutter, dipping cutter in flour between cuts. Place on ungreased baking sheet. Bake at 425° for 10 to 12 minutes. Makes 8 biscuits.

CARROTS WITH COCONUT

¼ cup flaked coconut
2 pounds carrots, cut crosswise in ¼-inch slices
2 tablespoons margarine or butter
1 teaspoon salt
½ teaspoon ground nutmeg

Sprinkle coconut evenly in an ungreased jelly roll pan (15½ x 10½ x 1 inch). Toast in a 350° oven until golden brown, 10 to 15 minutes (watch carefully). Place steamer basket in ½ inch of water in a saucepan; place carrots in basket, cover tightly, and heat to boiling. Reduce heat; steam until carrots are tender, 12 to 15 minutes. Toss carrots with margarine, salt, and nutmeg. Sprinkle with coconut.

FRIED ASPARAGUS

2 to 2½ pounds asparagus, peeled
Batter for deep frying
Oil for deep frying
Salt

Blanch the asparagus in boiling salted water for 2 to 3 minutes. Drain and dry the stalks. Dip the stalks, one by one, into the batter and deep fry in hot oil at 375° until the batter is golden and crisp. When done, drain the asparagus on paper towels. Sprinkle with salt and serve hot. A great snack.

FRIED CARROTS

5 or 6 medium carrots, sliced into ¼-inch rounds
Salt
2 tablespoons olive oil
1 tablespoon flour, seasoned with salt and pepper
1 cup unflavored yogurt (if you tolerate yogurt)
½ teaspoon caraway seeds

Parboil the carrots in salty water. When almost soft, drain and cool a little. Heat the oil in a skillet, toss the carrots in the seasoned flour, and then fry them until they are brown. Arrange the carrots in a warmed serving dish; heat the yogurt to lukewarm, pour over the carrots, and sprinkle with the caraway seeds.

GARLIC OKRA PICKLES

3 pounds okra
3 cups water
1 cup white grain-based vinegar
¼ cup pickling salt
2 cloves garlic, minced

Pack whole fresh okra into hot, clean pint jars. Combine remaining ingredients; bring to boiling. Slowly pour boiling liquid into jars, leaving ½-inch head space. Prepare lids according to manufacturer's directions. Wipe jar rim. Adjust lid. Process jars in boiling water bath for 5 minutes (start timing when water returns to boil). Makes 4 pints.

GRATED SAUTÉED ZUCCHINI

4 to 6 small zucchini
2 scallions
2 tablespoons olive oil or butter
¼ teaspoon dried dillweed
2 tablespoons chopped fresh parsley
Salt and pepper

Scrub but do not peel the zucchini. Grate in a food processor or with a hand grater, using the coarse side. Drain the grated zucchini in a colander for 10 minutes, pressing the liquid out from time to time with a spoon. Chop the scallions. Heat the oil or butter in a skillet; add the scallions and sauté. The moment they become translucent, add the grated zucchini and the dill. Stir-fry for 2 to 3 minutes, cooking over medium-high heat. Cover and cook for 1 to 2 minutes. Add the parsley, salt, and pepper just before serving and mix well. Serves 2.

HARVARD BEETS

1 8½-ounce can sliced beets
1 teaspoon sugar (if you tolerate sugar)
1 teaspoon cornstarch
⅛ teaspoon salt
2 tablespoons grain-based vinegar
1 tablespoon butter or margarine

Drain beets, reserving ¼ cup liquid. In saucepan, combine sugar, cornstarch, and salt. Stir in reserved liquid, vinegar, and butter. Cook, stirring constantly, until mixture is thickened and bubbly. Stir in beets. Cook until heated through.

JERUSALEM ARTICHOKES WITH PARSLIED CREAM SAUCE

1 pound Jerusalem artichokes
2 tablespoons butter
2 tablespoons flour
½ teaspoon salt
Dash white pepper
1 cup light cream or milk
3 cups finely snipped parsley

Wash, peel, and slice artichokes. In covered pan, cook artichokes in a small amount of boiling salted water until tender, about 10 minutes. Drain well. Melt butter; blend in flour, salt, and white pepper. Add cream or milk. Cook and stir until thickened and bubbly. Remove from heat. Stir in snipped parsley. Serve over artichokes. Makes 4 to 6 servings.

Difficult Recipes

OXTAIL-LEEK STEW

⅓ cup all-purpose flour
5 pounds oxtails, disjointed
¼ cup shortening
1 cup chopped onion
1 large carrot, quartered
1 medium turnip, peeled and quartered
2 cloves garlic, minced
Few sprigs parsley
1 bay leaf
3 cups beef stock
1 cup water
1½ cups sliced carrots
2 cups sliced leeks

Combine flour, 2 teaspoons salt, and dash pepper. Coat oxtails with flour mixture. In large Dutch oven, brown oxtails in hot shortening, turning often; drain off fat. Add onion, the quartered carrot, turnip, garlic, parsley, and bay leaf. Stir in beef stock and water. Bring to a boil; reduce heat. Cover and simmer until oxtails are almost tender, about 1½ hours. Remove and discard the cooked carrot, turnip, parsley, and bay leaf. Skim off fat. Return the mixture to boiling; reduce heat. Add 1 teaspoon salt and dash pepper. Simmer, covered, for 30 minutes. Add sliced carrots; simmer 10 minutes longer. Add leeks; simmer until vegetables are just tender, 10 to 15 minutes longer. Makes 6 to 8 servings.

VEGETABLE-BEEF POT PIE

1½ pounds boneless chuck, cut into 1-inch cubes
6 tablespoons margarine
1½ cup Lawry's or French's Brown Gravy Mix®
1½ cups thin carrot strips, 1 inch long
1 cup onion (chopped)
1 cup diced celery
1½ cup french- or kitchen-cut beans (drained and rinsed)
6 tablespoons flour
Salt and pepper
8-ounce package Pillsbury Crescent Rolls®

Heat oven to 350°. Brown meat in margarine. Add carrots, onions, celery, green beans, salt and pepper. Add gravy mix. Simmer 20 minutes. Add a little water, if needed. Combine flour with a little gravy; add back in and heat until thick. Pour in greased loaf pan (9 x 13). Unroll dough into two rectangles. On wax paper, overlap long edges and press to seal; press or roll dough to fit pan; cut small designs out of dough. Place dough over meat and vegetables. Decorate with cut out dough. Brush with beaten egg. Bake at 350° for 30 minutes until golden.

For the Wild at Heart

MARINATED VENISON IN CREAM GRAVY

4- to 5-pound venison roast, from leg if possible
1 cup chopped onion
⅓ cup oil
2 (12-ounce) cans beer
2 teaspoons salt
1 teaspoon thyme
8 peppercorns
2 garlic cloves, minced
1 bay leaf
½ cup cream or half and half
Flour

Place venison in large glass bowl. Sauté onion in oil. Stir in beer and seasonings and pour over venison. Marinate in refrigerator 24 hours, turning occasionally. Place venison and marinade in Dutch oven, cover, and bake at 325° for 2½ hours or until tender, basting several times. (May be cooked rare if from a young animal.)

Transfer meat to a platter. Strain liquid and skim off most of the fat. Measure liquid. Make a paste of cream and 2 tablespoons flour for each cup of liquid. Combine paste with liquid in sauce pan and cook, stirring constantly, until thickened. Season to taste. Two to 3 servings per pound.

GOOSE

When you prepare goose, here are a few tips to remember. Always roast the goose on a rack to allow the grease to drain. Try stuffing the goose with sauerkraut. It gives the bird and the kraut great flavor. Sprinkle the goose with paprika to aid in browning, just like a turkey.

WILD DUCK

Wash and clean ducks well; sprinkle cavity with salt and pepper, inside and out. Then place ¼ apple, celery stalks, and ¼ onion inside cavity (discard after cooking). Place in a roaster and bake slowly in 250° oven, approximately 2 to 3 hours. If cooked in too hot an oven, the duck will dry out.

STEWED RABBIT

2½ to 3 pounds rabbit
⅓ cup flour
1 teaspoon salt, divided
¼ teaspoon pepper
6 slices cut up bacon
1 large onion, sliced
2 med. carrots, cut crosswise into 12-inch slices
2 med. cloves garlic, crushed
1 bay leaf
1¼ cup water
1 tablespoon packed brown sugar
½ teaspoon dried rosemary leaves
½ teaspoon paprika
1 tablespoon cornstarch
2 tablespoons cold water

Cut rabbit into pieces. Mix flour, ½ teaspoon salt, and pepper; coat rabbit. Fry bacon in 4-quart Dutch oven until crisp. Remove bacon, drain, and reserve. Pour off all but 2 tablespoons of bacon fat. Cook rabbit in fat over medium heat, turning occasionally, until brown. Add onions, carrots, garlic, reserved bacon, and bay leaf. Mix 1¼ cup water, brown sugar, ½ teaspoon salt, rosemary, and paprika; pour over the rabbit. Heat to boiling; reduce heat, cover, and simmer until rabbit is tender, about 1 to 1½ hours. Remove rabbit and vegetables and keep warm. Mix cornstarch and 2 tablespoons cold water; stir into liquid in Dutch oven. Heat to boiling, stirring constantly. Boil and stir 1 minute. Pour sauce over rabbit and vegetables.

Bibliography

Abelson, P. H., Butz, E., and Snyder, S. H. *Neuroscience.* Washington, D.C.: American Association for the Advancement of Science, 1985.

Allen, D. H., Delohery, J., and Baker, G. "Monosodium L-Glutamate Induced Asthma," *Journal of Allergy and Clinical Immunology*, Vol. 80, 1987: pp. 530–7.

Allstetter, B., "Cheating Brain Death," *Discover*, Vol. 12, No. 8, August 1991: p. 24.

Bigelow, W. D., and Dunbar, P. B. "The Acid Content of Fruits," *Journal of Industrial and Engineering Chemistry*, Vol. 9, No. 8, August 1917: pp. 762–767.

Costa, E., and Greengard, P. *Advances in Biochemical Psychopharmacology, Volume 27, Glutamate as a Neurotransmitter.* New York: Raven Press, 1981.

Ebert, A. G. Letters to the Editor, *Journal of Asthma*, Vol. 20, No. 2, 1983: pp. 161–3.

Ensminger, A. H., Ensminger, M. E., Konland, E. K., and Robson, J. R. K. *Foods and Nutrition Encyclopedia.* Clovis, California: Pegus Press, 1983.

Fernandez-Flores, E., Kline, D. A., Johnson, A. R., and Leber, B. L. "Quantitative and Qualitative TLC Analysis of Free Amino Acids in Fruits and Fruit Juices," *Journal of the Association of Official Analytical Chemists*, Vol. 53, No. 6, 1970: pp. 1203–8.

Filer, L. J., Garattini, S., Kare, M. R., Reynolds, W. A., and Wurtman, R. J. (eds.) *Glutamic Acid: Advances in Biochemistry and Physiology*. New York: Raven Press, 1979.

Guidotti, A. *Fidia Research Foundation Symposium Series, Volume 4, Neurotoxicity of Excitatory Amino Acids*. New York: Raven Press, 1990.

Hac, L. R., Long, M. L., and Blish, M. J. "The Occurrence of Free L-Glutamic Acid in Various Foods," *Food Technology*, October 1949: pp. 351–4.

Kliewer, W. M. "Free Amino Acids and Other Nitrogenous Substances of Table Grape Varieties," *Journal of Food Science*, Vol. 34, 1969: pp. 274–8.

Leon, A. S., Hunninghake, D. B., Bell, C., Rassin, D. K., and Tephly, T. R. "Safety of Long-Term Large Doses of Aspartame," *Archives of Internal Medicine*, Vol. 149, October 1989: pp. 2318–24.

Maeda, S., Egushi, S., and Sasaki, H. "The Free L-Glutamic Acid Content of Foods (Report No. 2)," *Journal of Home Economics*, Vol. 12, No. 2, 1969: pp. 105–6.

Olney, J. W. "Brain Lesions, Obesity, and Other Disturbances in Mice Treated with Monosodium Glutamate," *Science*, Vol. 164, May 9, 1969: pp. 119–21.

Olney, J. W. "Brain Damage in Infant Mice Following Oral Intake of Glutamate, Aspartate, or Cysteine," *Nature*, Vol. 227, August 8, 1970: pp. 609–11.

Potenza, D. P., and El-Mallakh, R. S. "Aspartame: Clinical Update," *Connecticut Medicine*, Vol. 53, No. 7, July 1989: pp. 395–400.

Reinhardt, D., and Schmidt, E. *Nestle Nutrition Workshop Series, Volume 17, Food Allergy*. New York: Raven Press, 1988.

Robinson, A. L., "Neurotransmitters Regulate Growth Cones," *Science*, Vol. 234, December 12, 1986: pp. 1325–6.

Saravis, S., Schachar, R., Zlotkin, S., Leiter, L. A., and Anderson, G. H. "Aspartame: Effects on Learning, Behavior, and Mood," *Pediatrics*, Vol. 86, No. 1, July 1990: pp. 75–83.

Scopp, A. L. "MSG and Hydrolyzed Vegetable Protein Induced Headache: Review and Case Studies," *Headache*, Vol. 31, No. 2, February 1991: pp. 107–10.

Souci, S. W., Fachmann, W., and Kraut, H. *Food Composition and Nutrition Tables 1986/87*. Stuttgart, Germany: Wissenschaftliche Verlagsgesellshaft GmbH, 1986.

Steginck, L. D., Filer, L. J. *Aspartame: Physiology and Biochemistry*. New Yor, and Basel: Marcel Dekker, Inc., 1984.

Swan, G. F. Letters to the Editor, *Journal of Asthma*, Vol. 20, No. 2, 1983: pp. 159–61.

Wilkin, J. K., "Does Monosodium Glutamate Cause Flushing (Or Merely 'Glutamania')?" *Journal of the American Academy of Dermatology*, Vol. 15, 1986: pp. 225–30.

Wurtman, R. J., and Wurtman, J. J. *Nutrition and the Brain, Volume 6, Physiological and Behavioral Effects of Food Constituents*. New York: Raven Press, 1983.

Yost, D. A. "Clinical Safety of Aspartame," *American Family Physician*, Vol. 39, No. 2, February 1989: pp. 201–6.

Zautcke, J. L., Schwartz, J. A., and Mueller, E. J. "Chinese Restaurant Syndrome: A Review," *Annals of Emergency Medicine*, Vol. 15, No. 10, October 1986: pp. 1210–13.

NOTES

NOTES

NOTES

NOTES

ORDER FORM

To order by mail, complete and return this form (with payment) to the address below. To order by phone, call (612) 645-8182 (have your Mastercard/Visa information ready).

TITLE	QTY.	PRICE
Food Allergy Treatment, My Way ($9.95)	_____	_____
SHIPPING AND HANDLING (3rd Class)		$2.25
(Eliminate charge if you pick up book at our office.)		
SUBTOTAL		_____
SALES TAX (6.5%)		_____
(Minnesota residents only)		
TOTAL		_____

MAKE CHECKS PAYABLE TO: ACA Publications

CHARGE MY: ❑ VISA ❑ MASTERCARD

CARD NO. _____ EXPIRATION DATE_____

AUTHORIZED SIGNATURE _____

NAME _____

SHIPPING ADDRESS _____

CITY/STATE/ZIP_____

MAIL THIS FORM WITH PAYMENT TO:

ACA Publications
1690 University Avenue West, Suite 450
St. Paul, Minnesota 55104
(612) 645-8182

PLEASE ALLOW 4 WEEKS FOR DELIVERY